Biological Awareness:
Statements for Self-Discovery

Biological Awareness:

statements for self-discovery

D. W. Edington
University of Massachusetts

Lee Cunningham
Fitchburg State College

PRENTICE-HALL, Inc. *Englewood Cliffs, New Jersey*

Library of Congress Cataloging in Publication Data

EDINGTON, D   W   *Date*
    Biological awareness.

    Bibliography: p.
      1. Exercise—Physiological effect—Testing.
2. Exercise—Physiological effect—Study and
teaching. 3. Body, Human—Study and teaching
I. Cunningham, Lee, joint author. II. Title.
[DNLM: 1. Hormones—Physiology—Congresses.
2. Thymus gland—Physiology—Congresses. WK400
B615 1974]
QP301.E3   612'.76   75-16117
ISBN 0-13-077180-5

© 1975 by Prentice-Hall, Inc.

Printed in the United States of America.

10 9 8 7 6 5 4 3 2 1

PRENTICE-HALL INTERNATIONAL, INC., *London*
PRENTICE-HALL OF AUSTRALIA, PTY. LTD., *Sydney*
PRENTICE-HALL OF CANADA, LTD., *Toronto*
PRENTICE-HALL OF INDIA PRIVATE LIMITED, *New Delhi*
PRENTICE-HALL OF JAPAN, INC., *Tokyo*
PRENTICE-HALL OF SOUTHEAST ASIA (PTE.) LTD., *Singapore*

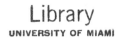

We would like to dedicate this book to our wives Marilyn and Marie; to our sons and daughter David Glen Edington, Scott Nelson Cunningham, and Cindy Lee Cunningham; and more especially to the teachers of physical education, exercise, and sport who will teach these and other young people about their bodies.

Contents

8 Energy Support Systems   183

Glossary   229

General Bibliography   235

Index   239

chapter 1

Introduction

Biological awareness can be defined as a full consciousness of one's body and knowledge of how it can respond to the demands of the environment. We believe that this awareness is important for the individual, and that it can be taught. In the words of Jerome Bruner, "There is no reason to believe that any subject cannot be taught to any child at virtually any age in some form."[1] To this end, then, we have developed a series of "statements" that encompass a conceptual approach to teaching biological awareness.

The lessons herein emphasize "self-discovery" experiments based on single focus sentences within various important categories related to biological functioning. They are designed to be given not as lectures requiring long periods of sitting and arousing student boredom, but as fast, hard-hitting sessions that are over in five to fifteen minutes. These lessons are not intended to be an end in themselves, but can be used as a supplement to the regular science or health class, as special class projects, or in regular physical education programs. Our concern is to make available understandable concepts that can be utilized by each student. These concepts are primarily intended to allow the

[1] *The Process of Education* (Cambridge, Mass.: Harvard University Press, 1961).

1

involved student to make good decisions regarding his or her body in future years. We stress that the success of an educational program should be judged by the lasting appropriateness of behavior and the present and future ability of the student to make rational decisions based on the best possible evidence.

Given the reevaluative thinking of preventive medicine and the projected advances in biology, including those advances in adaptative mechanisms to stress, disease, and aging, we think it is particularly imperative that school-age people be exposed to the way their bodies respond to stress. Because the public schools reach nearly 70 percent of the population of the United States, they are the obvious places to initiate programs that will allow human beings to discover, experience, and understand their bodies.

The "statements" in this text have been developed because we suspect that in all too many cases students (college as well as school-age) take biological and/or physiological science courses and thereafter proceed to utilize very little of what they have learned—probably because they simply do not see how to apply this information to their personal situations. These statements in this book allow students to discover biological responses through personal experience.

We feel that most qualified teachers have the necessary background to guide their students through these lessons. A partial physiological basis is provided for each statement and additional information can be gained by consulting the reference lists that are found at the end of the sections.

The model in Figure 1–1 shows the organization we have followed to systematically develop the appropriate statements. We have chosen to partition biological awareness into five primary categories—Orientation to Exercise, Somatology, The Neuromuscular System, Energy Systems, and Energy Support Systems.

The Orientation to Exercise category includes an exercise fitness profile and a description of the specificity of exercise theory. We are acutely concerned that people learn to appreciate the several different types of exercise.

The Somatology category emphasizes body composition and health-related areas including weight-control strategies. The purpose of this category is to heighten an awareness of body image and the control a person has over his or her own body.

In the Neuromuscular category, muscle function and control and motor learning are emphasized so that movement potentials and capabilities can be realized.

The Energy Systems and Energy Support Systems categories include statements that concentrate on the physiological limitations to exercise. Here the physiological mechanisms that operate during exer-

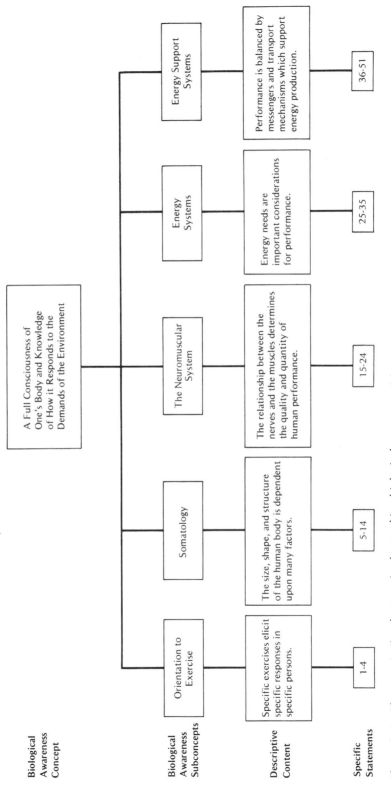

Biological Awareness Concept

A Full Consciousness of One's Body and Knowledge of How it Responds to the Demands of the Environment

Biological Awareness Subconcepts

| Orientation to Exercise | Somatology | The Neuromuscular System | Energy Systems | Energy Support Systems |

Descriptive Content

Specific exercises elicit specific responses in specific persons.

The size, shape, and structure of the human body is dependent upon many factors.

The relationship between the nerves and the muscles determines the quality and quantity of human performance.

Energy needs are important considerations for performance.

Performance is balanced by messengers and transport mechanisms which support energy production.

Specific Statements

1-4　5-14　15-24　25-35　36-51

Figure 1–1. The organizational categories for teaching biological awareness statements.

3

cise are explored, with demonstrations of the ways in which the body adapts to training as opposed to sedentary living.

We hope that this book will not only provide concrete examples for teaching but will serve as an innovative stimulus to the student

surrounding environment.

and/or teacher in the development of other statements in the interests of encouraging individuals to explore their bodies as related to the

chapter 2

Contemporary Curriculum Models and Biological Awareness

The contemporary school curriculum shows an increasing trend toward humanistic education. Theoretically, humanistic education provides for the maximum development of each student's academic potential and allows for greater teacher–pupil and pupil–pupil interaction. The biological awareness conceptual approach is one attempt to provide the physical education, health, or science instructor with the information for adaptation to an educational program that is individually guided.

Several models of physical education have been proposed; the purpose of this chapter is to refer to selected models and demonstrate the application of our biological awareness statements to each.

Evaul has proposed a model for curriculum construction in physical education involving the concept "Man Functions Through Movement."[1] He lists three subconcepts to expand this basic thought with several organizing centers from which instruction can be planned (Figure 2–1). He suggests that present-day physical education exists only in the third subconcept, "Movement Takes Many Forms." It is our con-

[1] Tom Evaul, "Where Are You Going? What Are You Going to Do?", paper presented at the Regional Conference for Curriculum Improvement in Secondary School Physical Education, Mt. Pocono, 1971.

5

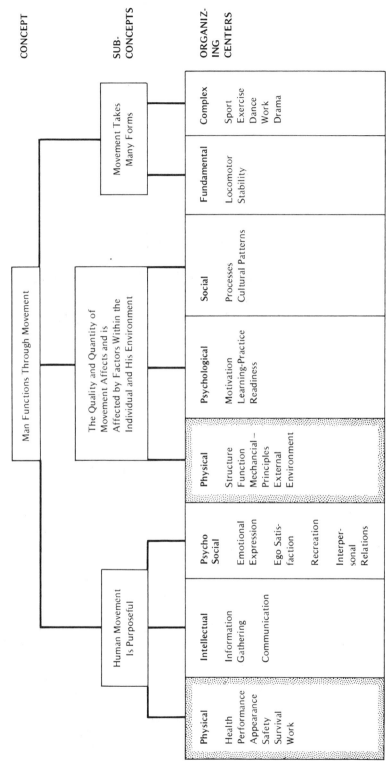

Figure 2–1. Evaul's proposed structure for the study of human movement. Reprinted by permission of author and AAHPER, Regional Conference for Curriculum Improvement in the Secondary School Physical Education, 1971.

tention, however, that the biological awareness approach can be applied to Evaul's first two subconcepts. Under the second subconcept, for example, many of the statements from Chapter 4 could be utilized. Imagine a unit in the schools applying Evaul's model and biological awareness statements entitled "Movement and Somatology," "Movement and the Nerve Muscle Relationship," "Movement and Preventive Medicine", or "Movement and the Internal Environment." This certainly would be a challenging and exciting teaching assignment.

Jewett's model (Figure 2–2) for the secondary school lists a "Physical Fitness Element" with several modules for which biological awareness lessons seem appropriate.[2] Lessons can be applied to the modules of muscular strength (Statements 16, 18), circulorespiratory endurance (Statements 30, 32, 33, 34, 37, 38, 39, 40), weight training (Statement 19), jogging (Statements 37, 38), and circuit training (Statement 20).

Johnson, in calling for a national model for physical education,[3] stresses the need for greater attention to the cognitive and affective domains as described by Bloom.[4] Currently, physical education instruction seems only to concentrate in the psychomotor domain with primarily incidental teaching. Johnson maintains that planned objectives in the cognitive and affective areas are a necessity for contemporary physical education. The biological awareness approach can provide lessons involving the cognitive domain of knowledge, apprehension, application, analysis, synthesis, and evaluation. Many of our statements internalize the results of the lessons by using values clarification strategies within the affective domain.

The Biological Science Curriculum Study (BSCS) group has developed a "Human Sciences Middle School Project" which integrates a variety of biosocial subjects.[5] An analysis of this project indicates a definite role for the physical educator and health educator utilizing biological awareness techniques in such content topics as stress, biochemical homeostasis, adaptation, nutrition, drugs, growth and development, locomotion, size-strength, sports, aging, and physical abilities. The point is, we must utilize our physical education expertise beyond the level of skill teaching. The content topic, "Physical Abilities," for example, could include our test and measurements materials. For years

[2]Ann E. Jewett, "Physical Education Objectives Out of Curricular Chaos," paper presented at the Regional Conferences for Curriculum Improvement in Secondary School Physical Education, Mt. Pocono, 1971.

[3]Perry Johnson, "Is There A Need for A National Model for School Physical Education?", paper presented at the AAHPER Convention in Minneapolis, April 1973.

[4]Benjamin S. Bloom, ed., *Taxonomy of Educational Objectives Handbook: Cognitive Domain* (New York: David McKay Co., Inc., 1956).

[5]Human Sciences: A Development Approach to Adolescent Education. Biological Science Curriculum Study, Boulder, Colorado, 1973.

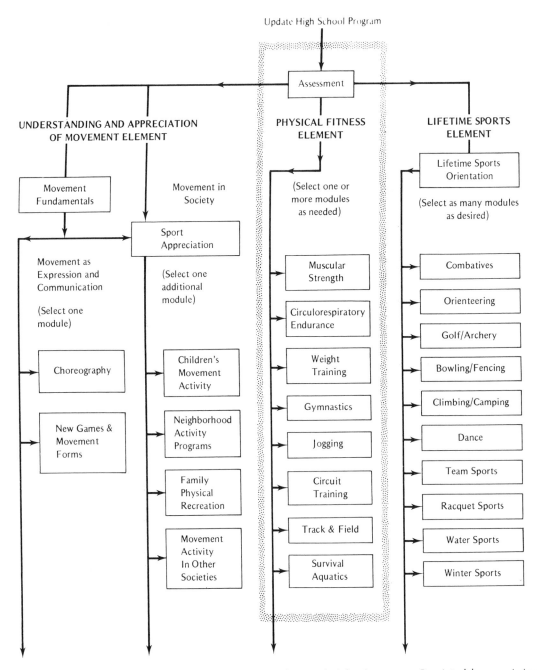

Figure 2–2. Jewett's Physical Education Objective: Update High School program. Reprinted by permission of author and AAHPER, Regional Conference for Curriculum Improvement, 1971.

8

physical fitness tests have been administered with only a small portion of the educational value of such tests being utilized. What is the physical ability tested by the 50-yard dash? We test the student, give a percentile score, and then never discuss it again. Does size, height, weight, leg girth measurements, or strength relate to this speed component? How does this differ according to age and sex? A discussion of other physical abilities such as strength, agility, coordination, reaction time, flexibility, etc., can be undertaken through the medium of performance evaluation. Vander Zwaag,[6] in discussing the seven distinguishing characteristics of sport points out that each activity has physical attributes that contribute to performance. This would make for an excellent learning experience relating biological awareness and sport theory. These are examples of the type of thinking necessary in the integrative curriculum. Statements 23 and 24 are appropriate to this area.

Burnstine has proposed a physical education curriculum for the Glen Ridge, N.J. High School.[7] She includes a mini-lab course in basic concepts of physical activity (e.g., strength, fitness, flexibility, skill learning, and weight control) for the tenth and eleventh grades as a part of the curriculum design (Figure 2–3). This Burnstein curriculum could utilize most of the biological awareness statements proposed in this text.

Because many high schools are developing new and different courses, particularly in the eleventh and twelfth years of school, exercise physiology on that level is a reality. Meyers has recently described a program developed in West Hartford, Connecticut.[8] The course is a formal half-year approach to exercise physiology using the lecture and laboratory technique.

Because of limited equipment budgets in most schools, the experiments discussed in this text may be readily applied. Only a small initial outlay of money can equip a high school with a limited but effective health and fitness laboratory.

Our proposed model is a physical education curriculum continuum that can be applied to grades K–12 (Table 2–1). Although each level should have different objectives, biological awareness is an integral part of each grade category. The biological awareness objective as shown is wedge-shaped to allow for greater in-depth study as the students' cognitive abilities develop.

[6]Harold J. Vander Zwaag, "Distinguishing Characteristics of Sport." Proceedings, 77th Annual Meeting, National College Physical Education Association for Men. 11:70–78, 1974.

[7]Diedre Burnstine, "On Considering Curriculum Design," paper presented at AAHPER Regional Conference for Curriculum Improvement in Secondary School Physical Education, Mt. Pocono, 1971.

[8]Edward Meyers, "Exercise Physiology in Secondary Schools: A Three Dimensional Approach. *Journal of Health, Physical Education and Recreation* 46:30–31, 1975.

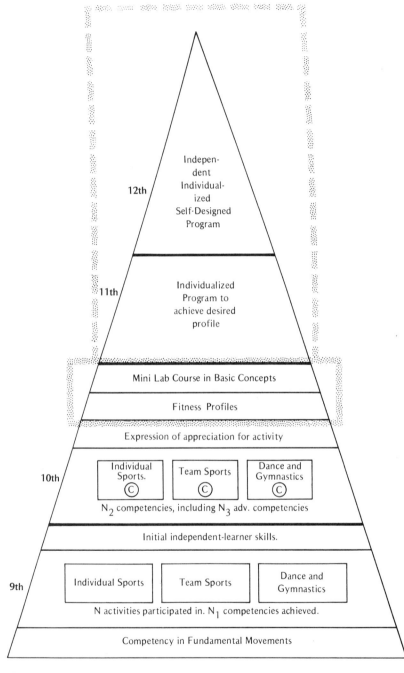

Figure 2–3. Burnstine's model of proposed physical education curriculum for Glen Ridge High School. Reprinted by permission of author and AAHPER, Regional Conference for Curriculum Improvement, 1971.

The K–3 program must be movement-experiential and perceptual-motor in nature. The child should learn how the body responds to different forces, movements, directions, and objects. The physical education instructor can incorporate biological awareness through simple lessons in balance, flexibility, directionality, strength, coordination, endurance, agility, etc. For example, a lesson on balance might include the directions to balance "as high as possible," "as low as possible," "while moving," "on only one point," "with your eyes shut," "on an object," "an object," "with a partner"; also, the instructor might ask, "How many different types of balance can you think of?" A lesson using movement exploration applied to flexibility might include such questions as "Can you bend your body?" "a different part of your body?" "in a different direction?" "How far can you bend your arms, legs, hands, feet, and body?" "Can you bend more than two parts at the same time? in opposite direction?" etc.

With lessons such as these children can experience and discover the concepts of balance and flexibility. This will prepare them for an understanding of these two components for sports participation, which is the next objective in our continuum. The middle school child can begin to understand flexibility and balance related to organized play. What role does flexibility and balance play in learning a new sports skill? Do different sports require different amounts of balance and flexibility? How do you train for flexibility and balance? What activities promote flexibility and balance?

The senior high school curriculum will allow the student to study balance in greater depth, perhaps evaluating the types of tests to assess balance, administer balance tests to others, and even to examine the vestibular apparatus that is involved in balance. Flexibility studies can involve studying the anatomy of the joint, more sophisticated assessment techniques, athletic injuries, and rehabilitation.

TABLE 2-1. The Cunningham-Edington Physical Education Curriculum continuum.

	K	1	2	3	4	5	6	7	8	9	10	11	12
Movement Experiences and Perceptual-Motor Skills	▭												
Sports Education					▭								
Lifetime Sports and Recreation										▭			
Biological Awareness Statements	◁▭▭▭▭▭▭▭▭▭▭▭▷												

If perceptual-motor and movement experiences are the objectives in K–3, then it may be important in grades 4–6 to integrate some fundamental movements in a more disciplined fashion. Sports education may be taught at this age level. Physiologically and developmentally, children of this age are ready to perform higher skills. We must not only provide for objectives in the psychomotor domain, but work with the affective and cognitive domains as well. Our goals must be more than incidental. In teaching sports for children we must develop a sensitivity toward the aim of the activity, the rules, strategy, teammate relationships, opponents, the coach, winning, and losing. Sportsmanship should be rediscovered. We are dealing with a medium for the development of humanistic values through sports. This idea should be central to the curriculum in grades 4–6, and not merely the development of players for future interscholastic athletics.

In the upper middle school years, grades 7 and 8, it is time to perfect performance in sports. There should be a solid basis in the elementary program of movement education and elementary skills that have been taught in a more thoughtful manner in grades 4–6. The upper middle school is a time for perfecting these skills through activity. Individual and team sports can be continued and lifetime sports should be introduced. However, we must be careful not to include activities that will be overlapped in the high school years.

Biological awareness is important to students of this age. Both boys and girls are receptive to hints about their bodies and training. Owing to the unevenness in growth, girls at this stage are extremely figure-conscious. Biological awareness lessons in diet and nutrition and the effects of exercise on body composition must be planned. The boys characteristically are smaller than the girls and they often show interest in body configuration. A properly presented weight training program for muscle development is important at this stage.

Grade 9–12 are vital years, providing our last chance to influence activity patterns in the school-age population. At least 70 percent of our students are not touched by formal activity programming after grade 12, so these years are important in integrating physical activity into the lifestyle of young people. We must deal with the scientific principles of activity. Although it is important to plan for cognitive and affective objectives through principles of exercise throughout the entire spectrum of K–12, it becomes particularly vital to deal with biological awareness in the high school program.

Grades 9–12 are important in recreational sports, outdoor activities, and lifetime sports. Preventive medicine can be a theme during this period of time, including a study of the values of exercise and its application to health.

We have attempted to illustrate that the biological awareness approach has application to several contemporary educational curricula. The effectiveness of such application is dependent upon the creativity, adaptability, and enthusiasm of the classroom teachers. Chapter 3 will discuss the utilization of this approach, including how our statements can be adapted to various grade levels, how biological awareness statements may be created, and will give some examples of how to adapt these statements.

Utilization of Biological Awareness Statements

The question now arises, "How do I use biological awareness information in my situation?" Our answer is, "However you see fit."

With that as an introduction, several possibilities for utilization of this information can be offered. The first point to remember is that the "cookbook" approach is doomed to failure from the outset because it does not allow for teacher creativity or enthusiasm. If a particular statement fits your instructional needs, by all means use it, but do not start at Statement 1 and go to 51 and expect an educational miracle. Instead, each lesson should be adapted according to the age of the students, the topic under discussion, the class to which the material is being taught, the philosophy of the school, the attitude of the students, the equipment available, the time available, etc.

The biological awareness approach can be utilized by several academic disciplines: health, physical education, science, home economics, or some type of integrative approach. It can be used not only in the schools, but in recreational centers, in summer camps, at the YMCA; it can also be adapted to middle-aged and aging adults. Although this particular set of statements is most appropriate for use at the level of the secondary school and college foundations courses, with the appropriate adaptation they can easily be used with more mature adults or in the middle school (grades 4–8).

The method for utilization of the biological awareness statements suggested in this book is dependent upon the course, school, time available, curriculum, the value placed on this approach by the instructor, and the student population. Some suggested approaches would include:

Single Courses in Health or Physical Education

Many colleges are teaching courses in Exercise, Health, and Fitness to freshman as a general physical education requirement. It is our opinion that half- or full-year courses such as "Health and Fitness," "Movement and Health," "Foundations of Physical Activity," or "Introduction to Biological Fitness" can be offered on the secondary school level as well.

Mini-Lessons in a Regular Physical Education Class

Select one topic a week from the statements listed in this book and adapt it to a fifteen-minute mini-lesson. This lesson should not be boring, but quick and hard-hitting with some visual aids and bulletin board materials. For example, Statement 18—*Muscle strength is related to the length of the muscle at the time of contraction*—can be presented simply through several stick drawings on the locker-room bulletin board depicting the strength of the biceps through the range of forearm flexion (Figure 3–1).

If you were to lift a heavy weight, at what angle
would you have the greatest strength?

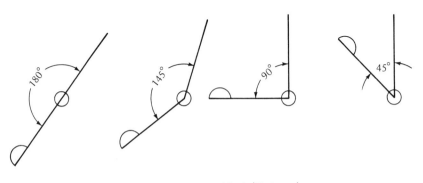

Which is the strongest position? (Circle one)

A   B   C   D

Figure 3–1. A possible "Theme for the Week"

Every year several specific health problems have a "national" week. We suggest that the statement appropriate to that health condition be used during that week. For example, during Diabetes Week the topic would come from Statement 45 (Insulin and Exercise).

Special Situations

How many days does it rain when the physical education class is supposed to go outside? How many days during the school year is the gym in use for special events such as art shows, preparation for a dance, pep rallies, and special assembly programs? You have eighty students split among three teachers with only two teaching stations; the third group has the locker room, corridor, or cafeteria. How about biological awareness lessons for such circumstances?

The Biological Awareness-Fitness Laboratory Concept

Although space is a problem in most school settings, with some creative thinking a location could be set aside for fitness-related materials, exercise equipment, assessment devices, and program materials. Many high schools have advanced science courses. With such a laboratory available it might be possible to integrate exercise physiology into the science curriculum.

Exercise Physiology Course in Colleges and High Schools

Although we realize that most college exercise physiology courses go far beyond the scope of the biological awareness exercises contained in this book, their practical application is oftentimes overlooked. Biological awareness concepts could be used in conjunction with exercise physiology to provide experiences to those who may someday teach these concepts. Far too many prospective teachers and coaches take a good course in exercise physiology and then proceed to apply very little of it in the future years. Part of the explanation for this may be that most people see very few ways to readily adapt the concepts from exercise physiology to their own situation.

Exercise physiology is now being included in many high school physical education curricula. The laboratory portion is ready-made using selected statements from this book.

Individual Guided Education (IGE)

IGE breaks from the traditional approach in that, although still structured, the student can progress at his or her own rate and materials can be selected that are interesting to individual students. Most of the materials in the text can be adapted into an IGE package which would be available to the student in a fitness or health module.

How to Create a Biological Awareness Statement

Our technique for creating a biological awareness statement[1] is outlined in Table 3–1. To illustrate how this technique may be applied to a specific situation, we have selected a highly scientific fitness or health concept and developed it into a teachable statement. For the sake of discussion we have developed the following statement for a fifth-grade class.

A. List the statement to be taught.

We decided to illustrate the scientific statement, *The muscle cell is a highly organized and specialized cell with connections to the nervous and cardiovascular systems.* The performance objective was stated as

---

TABLE 3–1.   How to Develop a Biological Awareness Statement

A. List the statement to be taught.
1. What are its performance objectives?
2. Is it relevant?
3. Is it appropriate for the grade and age level?
4. Is it integrated with the established teaching progression?
B. State the physiological basis of the statement.
1. Is it scientifically accurate in light of recent research and professional consensus?
2. Is it simple and understandable?
C. Develop the technique for teaching the statement.
1. Is it small, simple, and uncomplicated?
2. Can the students learn by performing some activity related to the statement?
3. Can a partner or team approach be used?
4. Is it in harmony with the stated performance objectives?
5. Is the desired outcome easily measured?
6. What is the best method for teaching this statement?
7. What alternatives are available for presenting the statement?
8. What equipment and materials are necessary to carry out this statement?
D. Develop some discussion questions to reinforce learning.
1. Create obvious answers.
2. Develop questions from the "physiological basis" of the statement and from the experience itself.

---

[1]See D. W. Edington, and Lee Cunningham, "More on Applied Physiology of Exercise," Journal of Health, Physical Education and Recreation, 45 (February 1974), 18.

follows: The student should be able to experientially simulate a molecule of food and/or oxygen which is transported by the cardiovascular system and undergoes change in the muscle cell in response to a message from the nervous system." We suggest that this difficult lesson can be illustrated by the use of a short "movement" playlet.

Is this lesson appropriate to the grade level and age of the child? From Chapter 1, to quote Bruner, "There is no reason to believe that any subject cannot be taught to any child at virtually any age in some form." It is clear that we must make the language appropriate to our fifth-grade class. Does it integrate with the present physical education, health, or science curriculum? It is our opinion that if education is to prepare young children with the scientific knowledge necessary for an understanding of life and health in the 1980s and 1990s, such statements about the body's response to stress are crucial to a totally educated person.

B. State the physiological basis of the statement.

(The following is an example of presenting this to the fifth-grade students.)

What gives the muscle the signal to move? What brings it the energy for the desired movement? Will the muscle stop if the signal and the delivery systems fail to meet the needs during hard activity such as bicycling or tree climbing?

The muscle needs fuel for the production of energy, mainly in the form of sugar and fat. This is similar to an automobile, which gets its energy from its fuel—gasoline. For the energy-releasing fuel to be burned, oxygen from the air we breathe is necessary. Likewise, the automobiles fuel needs oxygen to be burned. Fuel and oxygen, then, are extremely important for the production of energy—to turn the wheels in the automobile and to enable the body to move. But how do the fuel and oxygen get to the muscle in the body and to the motor in the engine? The body has vessels that are connected to the muscles that carry the materials pumped by the heart. Can you suggest how the gasoline gets to the engine in a car? The nervous system will tell the body what to do once enough energy is available. Thus the heart and vessels, and the nerves and the muscles must work together as a team if we are to move.

C. Develop the technique for teaching the statement.

The particular technique chosen to illustrate this statement involving the relationship originally stated between the nervous system, the cardiovascular system, and the muscle cells is a playlet. The students should imagine they are oxygen molecules being carried through the circulatory system, to the muscle cells. They become oxygen molecules in the lungs, then travel to the muscles where they undergo change to energy molecules. As energy molecules they then perform movement in response to a message from the nervous system (e.g., push-ups, forward roll, crawl, hop on one foot, etc.).

Using this type of playlet, the child may be able to get a feel for, and an understanding of, how muscle metabolism works and the interrelationship of the nervous and circulatory systems. To illustrate the rate of metabolism at rest or during levels of low energy demand, the actions should be performed slowly at first. Then, to show how these relationships adapt during high energy demands, the speed may be increased. Figure 3–2 presents a diagram of the suggested structure for conducting this lesson.

D. Develop some discussion questions to reinforce learning.

Ask some of the following questions: What did it feel like to be a molecule? How did it feel in the muscle cell? Do you suppose an actual molecule feels this way? What did the nervous system say to the muscle? Can you exercise so fast that the circulation and nervous systems cannot keep up with the demands? What happens?

This lesson can be structured directly into an elementary school physical education class. Obstacle courses including such activities as this playlet can be developed in many programs simply by adapting this example and slightly changing the objective to include more ac-

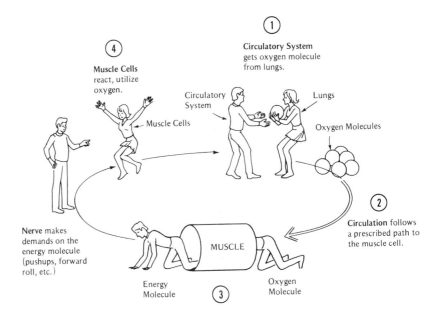

Figure 3–2. Muscle metabolism playlet for a 5th grade class.

tivity. This can be fun and can be accomplished without eliminating the physical activity that is so important.

How to Adapt Statements for Other Uses

As previously mentioned, these statements are suggested activities for use in the secondary school. This section will illustrate how they have been used or can be used at the elementary school, or secondary school and college level of general physical education, and for biological fitness.

Elementary School

The following four examples from Miganowicz[1] of "Why Exercise?" mini-lessons illustrate how the statements presented in this book have actually been adapted for grades 4–6.

Example 1. (Adapted from statements 40, 42) To show that during exercise the heart will work harder.

LESSON: Determination of pulse rate.

PROCEDURES
1. Show how to take pulse rate.
2. Take a resting pulse rate.
3. Exercise, then take another pulse rate.

DISCUSSION
Reasons for the increase? Will the heart become stronger?

FOLLOW-UP ACTIVITIES
Exercise could be shown to improve the cardiovascular system.

Example 2. (Adapted from Statements 30, 32, 38) To show (1) immediate effects of exercise; and (2) the difference between a student in "good" physical condition and one who is not.

LESSON: Observation of the body's responses before and after exercise; comparison of degrees of physical fitness.

PROCEDURES
1. The student runs or exercises vigorously.
2. Observe the immediate effects of exercise.
3. Discuss results.
   a. Respiratory rate, heart rate, pain in side, perspiration, etc.
   b. Differences—fitness

[1]William Miganowicz, "Applied Exercise Physiology in the Elementary School." A paper presented to the Massachusetts Association of HPER. April, 1972.

Example 3. (Adapted from Statements 37, 42, 43) To increase the cardiorespiratory rate.

LESSON: To show the relationship between the two systems and how they act under the stress of exercise.

PROCEDURES
1. Prepare a "body track." A student can trace the cardiac cycle and body scheme with a dump truck. The truck will move slowly showing the body at rest, then speed up according to increased energy demands.
2. Trace an outline of the heart and lungs on the floor or outdoor space. The students, acting as red blood cells, can move through the cardiac cycle. Once an understanding of the cycle has been achieved, each student can be "given" a molecule of oxygen when he reaches the lungs, for delivery somewhere in the body. He must exchange the oxygen for a carbon dioxide molecule, then return to the heart via the circulatory system, where the reverse exchange occurs.

Example 4. (Adapted from Statements 5, 6, 9, 26) To make certain alterations in the composition of your body.

LESSON: Somatotyping.

PROCEDURES
1. Display pictures of the three basic body types.
2. Describe the characteristics of each.
3. Discuss
   a. Activity limitations
   b. Possibility of making certain alterations through exercise and diet
   c. Individual body types and what can be done about them

FOLLOW-UP ACTIVITIES
Demonstrate certain activities.

Secondary School or College

The following are three examples of lecture outlines used by one of the authors in a lecture-laboratory course entitled Health and Fitness. The statements are integrated into the lecture portion to show the reader the lecture-laboratory relationship. With only slight modification, these outlines, with interrelated statements, can be used on the high school level.

Example 1. The intracellular environments, functions, and the training adaptations of muscle.

           i. Spinal cord
           ii. Pons
           iii. Midbrain
           iv. Cortex

3. Kinesthetic Sense
   a. Definition
   b. Components
      i. Perception of movement
      ii. Perception of tension
      iii. Balance (Statement 23)
      iv. Orientation in space
   c. spirokinesis (Statement 22)
4. The effects of drugs on the nervous system
5. Motor learning (Statement 24)

Example 3. Cardiovascular function and heart disease.

I. The anatomy of a heart attack.
   A. Heart and coronary vessels
   B. Vessels and microcirculation
   C. Types of coronary heart disease
      1. Coronary thrombosis and myocardial infarction
      2. Angina pectoris
      3. Stroke
      4. Hypertension (Statement 49)
   D. Stages of plaque development
      1. Lipid infiltration
      2. Fibrosis
      3. Calcium—cholesterol
   E. Etiology
      1. Statement 50
      2. Others
         a. Stress
         b. Urban living
         c. Churchgoing
         d. Socioeconomic status
         e. Radios, coffee
II. Cardiac intervention.
   A. Dietary modification
      1. Lipids—cholesterol and triglycerides
      2. Diets low in animal (unsaturated) fat and cholesterol
         a. Polyunsaturated to saturated fat ratio
         b. Diet studies

I. The muscle is a highly organized and speciali
   tions to the nervous and cardiovascular system
   A. The scheme of skeletal muscle
   B. The ultrastructure of a muscle cell
   C. The structure of a muscle fiber
   D. The contraction of skeletal muscle fibers—
   E. Types of muscle contractions

II. Exercise can be classified as a function of the
    upon the body and how the body responds to
    A. Classification of exercise—orientation to
       1. Speed and time considerations
       2. Speed and resistance considerations
       3. Resistance and time considerations
       4. Speed, time, and resistance considerat
    B. Specificity of exercise
       1. Skeletal muscle adapts differently to
          types of training demands:
          a. Low tension, high repetition (Stat
          b. High tension, low repetition (Sta
       2. Principles of training—overload and
          (Statement 19, 20)
    C. Training adaptations in skeletal muscle
       1. Hypertrophy
       2. Increased tone
          a. recruitment of motor units
          b. increased motor unit firing
          c. inhibition and facilitation
       3. Increased vascularization
       4. Alteration of fiber types
          a. Fast twitch
          b. Slow twitch

Example 2. Neuromuscular relationships.

I. The muscle cell will not function witho
   nervous system.
   A. The central nervous system and move
   B. The nerve-muscle relationship—motor
   C. Facilitation—inhibition

II. Neural control is important to human m
    A. Perceptual-motor integration
       1. Kephart
       2. Dowan-Delcato
          a. Sequence of motor developmen

B. Exercise prescription
  1. CV training effects/adaptions
    a. Blood composition
    b. Vascular integrity
    c. Increased tissue quality
    d. HR alterations (Statement 42)
    e. Increased output (Statement 43)
    f. Coronary artery improvement (Statement 50)
  2. How to start a cardiovascular training program
    a. See a doctor: check contraindications
    b. Relative fitness evaluation: health and fitness
      i. Percent body fat (Statement 6)
      ii. Flexibility (Statement 15)
      iii. Vital capacity (Statement 36)
      vi. Muscular strength and muscular endurance (Statements 16, 17, 18)
      v. Motor ability components: speed, agility, RT balance, power, steadiness (Statement 23)
      vi. Cardiovascular endurance (Statements 37, 38, 39)
    c. Four principles for developing a cardiovascular-aerobic program (Statement 39)
      i. Activities
      ii. Frequency (Statement 42)
      iii. Duration (Statement 38)
      iv. Intensity (Statements 41, 42)

Biological Fitness Programs

Biological awareness can be used as an approach to fitness assessment and programming. We do not intend to offer a new definition of fitness or create any new fitness dimensions, however; our approach is to unite fitness definitions, criteria, assessment techniques, and programming methods into one inclusive concept called *biological awareness.*

People uninformed   *People informed*
about their body   *about their body*

BIOLOGICAL AWARENESS CONTINUUM

All people fall somewhere on the biological awareness continuum. A world class champion in weight lifting, distance runner or swimmer, an exercise physiologist, or a physician who is involved in cardiac rehabilitation are some examples of people who would fall in the right half of the continuum (i.e., they would know something about the body and how it responds to the environment). The aim of the biological awareness statements is to bring about a shift in the knowledge base of the population to the right of the biological awareness continuum.

The decade of the 1950s was considered the "fitness era" in the development of physical education. Is our population in better condition now as a result of the emphasis placed on fitness in our schools during that time? What type of fitness education will be needed for the 1980s and 1990s? The goal of the biological awareness approach is to allow people to make intelligent choices about physical activity; they should be able to choose what is important to them about fitness, how to assess it, and how to program for it.

A new direction in the assessment of fitness is needed. If the student is to utilize the knowledge of how fast he can run the 50-yard dash, he must have some knowledge of the implications of speed. The biological awareness approach would make this possible. Furthermore, an evaluation of this parameter would be important as a guidance tool. Although the 50-yard dash seems to be an acceptable test to assess speed in professional sports, what of high school or college students who have no desire to become professional athletes? Must they be subjected to a speed test year after year with the hope that this parameter will be improved?

Biological awareness is then a process through which the student can learn about his or her body and its response to the environment. Finding out how well he or she performs various activities is useful, but only in developing the *process*, never as an end in itself.

What does all this mean in terms of biological awareness and fitness? This approach can sensitize the individual through a series of fitness and motor performance tests to his or her potential for success in a variety of activities. This means, however, that once an assessment has been made and interpreted there is little justification for retesting unless the student decides certain parameters to be important to his or her own relative fitness profile (Statement 4). This approach also allows the student to make some value decisions that are experientially based from the statements used. The *relative fitness profile* is provided to make exactly this choice of what seems to be important in terms of a personalized health and fitness program.

The integration of fitness considerations into the lifestyles of students should be an important goal. To make fitness a viable concept of education, however, requires an enthusiastic approach. We must spend less time stressing and practicing skills and more time emphasizing, through these skills, how the body works and how it responds to the demands of the environment.

chapter 4

Orientation to Exercise

statement **1**

Exercise can be classified as a function of the nature of the specific demands upon the body.

Introduction   To differentiate between the various types of exercises, a classification scheme is needed. Exercises are specific to the *speed* of movement, the *resistance* of that movement, and to the *duration of time* over which that movement has to be repeated.

Figure 4–1 shows that the faster the speed of movement, the shorter the time that exercise can be maintained; and conversely, the lower the speed of movement, the longer the exercise can be performed. For example, maximum running speed can be maintained for only a few seconds, while a much slower speed can be maintained for longer periods of time, such as in marathon competition.

Figure 4–2 indicates the relationship between the speed of movement and the resistance to that movement. For example, it is possible to move the arm faster when throwing a baseball (low resistance) than when throwing a shotput (higher resistance).

Figure 4–3 illustrates the resistance to movement and total exercise time (duration). Weightlifting exercises involving heavy weights can only be performed for a short period, while those same activities, if the weight (resistance) is reduced, can be maintained for an extended period of time.

Training of the proper intensity can shift that curve to the right in each of the three movement classifications, thus illustrating the role of training in performance.

A more complete classification would be to develop a three-dimensional construct (Figure 4–4). Although highly theoretical at this time, several uncomplicated activities can be located. This scheme for the classification of exercises can include a wide variety of activities (see teaching hints for illustrations). It must be remembered that biological awareness is defined as an understanding of the body and how the body responds to exercise demands. This statement should allow the student to graphically depict the different types of exercises.

Procedure   1. The student should place the following activities on the speed-duration chart.

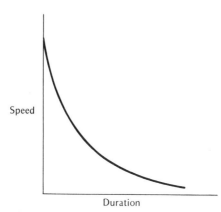

1. A 50-yd dash
2. 220-yd dash
3. ¼-mi run
4. 1-mi run
5. The 12-min or 1.5 mi aerobics test
6. 5-mi road race
7. 26-mi marathon

Figure 4–1.

2. Place the following activities on the speed-resistance chart:

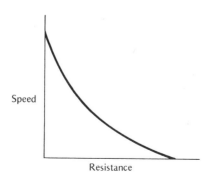

Arm speed in throwing a:
1. Ping-pong ball
2. Baseball
3. 16-lb shot put
4. 35-lb hammer
5. 1 repetition maximum (RM) in the bench press low or zero speed

Figure 4–2.

3. Place the following activities on the resistance-duration chart:

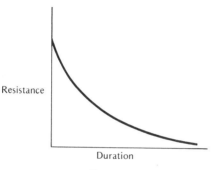

1. 1 RM for the bench press
2. Circuit weight training
3. Swimming ½ mi in 20 min
4. 8-hr walk on level ground

Figure 4–3.

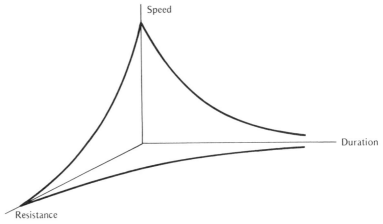

Figure 4–4. Classification scheme for physical activity including speed, duration, and resistance components.

Teaching Methods

Performance Objective

The student should be able to plot activities on the given charts based on the classification of speed, duration, and resistance.

Teaching Hints
1. See Procedures for activities and placements on the two-dimensional charts. (The activities are listed such that they are placed from upper left to lower right on the respective figures.)
2. The instructor should discuss this placement, then organize the students either individually or in small groups to plot a variety of activities (such as marathon running, 100-yd dash, competitive rowing, baseball, etc.) on the three-dimensional chart to show the relative contribution of speed, resistance and duration for a variety of activities.

Discussion
1. List your two favorite sports.
2. Plot both on Figures 4–1, 4–2, 4–3 and 4–4.
3. What type of training program must you undergo to shift your curves to the right in figures 4–2, 4–3 and 4–4.
4. What are the effects of training upon speed, resistance, and duration?
5. After performing some different exercises, can you tell what is a good indicator of exercise specificity? (Answer: muscle soreness.)

statement 2

Introduction   A specific exercise will elicit a specific response in a specific individual at a specific point in time. This implies that the end result of exercise is directly determined by each specific activity. Therefore, a knowledge of the specific details of the situation is essential in order to prescribe the correct set of activities to meet a given goal of an individual. "You get what you train for" is an exercise axiom that may be one of the most important concepts in the development of biological fitness.[1]

Exercise is specific to the biological system stressed, and when applied to the criteria of health and fitness and motor performance discussed in Statement 4, an evaluation of various activities can be made. For example, these criteria can be used to assess the contribution a specific activity makes to the biological system affected. By assigning the value of 0 for none, 1 for some, 2 for moderate, and 3 for maximum, each activity can be evaluated and compared for its specific potential for developing the desired fitness and/or performance criteria (see Table 4–1).

What activity would be considered the best for the promotion of total fitness?

List those activities which promote muscular strength.

List those activities which promote CV endurance.

List those criteria from the above table that are important to you.

Procedure   Using the chart provided, the student should list several activities and evaluate these in terms of the potential for development of specific fitness criteria.

Teaching Methods   *Performance Objective*

The student should be able to list several activities and evaluate each in terms of the suggested criterion.

[1]W. B. McCafferty and D. W. Edington, "The Subcellular Basis of Swimming." *Swimming Technique*, 10 (1974), 109–11.

TABLE 4–1.   Specificity Ratings of Selected Activities

ACTIVITY	CV Capacity	Flexibility	Muscular Strength	Muscular Endurance	Body Composition	Coordination	Agility	Power	Balance	Reaction Time	Speed
Jogging	3	1	1	1	2	1	1	0	1	0	1
Weight Training	1	2	3	1	2	1	0	2	1	2	0
White Water Canoeing	2	2	1	1	1	1	1	1	1	1	1

Teaching Hints
1. The evaluation of criteria is so subjective that agreement will be impossible.
2. Form small groups of students who will each evaluate the same activities. Have a feedback session of the evaluated activity and calculate the mean score for each criteria. A profile of several activities can be obtained.

Discussion   Develop a list of activities for the appropriate health and fitness criteria (jogging, basketball, tennis, bicycling would probably all be evaluated "3" in terms of cardiovascular (CV) capacity).

statement 3

> **The source of the chemical energy used for muscular work is dependent upon the intensity and duration of the exercise condition.**

Introduction There are primarily three biochemical sources of energy for human performance: (1) immediate sources, (2) nonoxidative sources, and (3) oxidative sources.[1] All fuel from these sources is utilized during specific time periods for the production of energy.

Time period I, as shown in Table 4–2 and Figure 4–5, involves any activity of less than one second; the energy comes from the ATP located on the contractile elements (the actin and myosin). The second period is also very short, providing the energy requirements for up to 10 seconds. In this period ATP formation is linked to the breakdown of creatine-phosphate, which is stored in the muscle during resting conditions.

Period III is a transitional time between short-term activity and that which might be considered nonoxidative. The energy for period IV, from 30 seconds to 2 minutes, is obtained from the nonoxidative breakdown of stored glycogen in the muscle. Lactate production is

TABLE 4–2. Time-Energy Source Chart

PERIOD	TIME INTERVAL	ENERGY SOURCE
I	less than one sec	Contractile elements and/or neural innervation
II	0 to 10 sec	ATP and creatine phosphate
III	10 to 30 sec	Transition
IV	30 sec to 2 min	Nonoxidative (glycogen)
V	2 to 5 min	Transition
VI	more than 5 min	Oxidative (glycogen and fat)

[1]D. W. Edington and V. Reggie Edgerton, *Biology of Activity* (Boston: Houghton-Mifflin Co., 1976.)

35

commonly observed during these types of exercise stresses. Another transition period, period V, lasts from 2 to about 5 minutes as the muscle begins to get a significant amount of energy from the direct utilization of oxygen.

The final period (VI) is for long-term exercise, deriving energy from the oxidative breakdown of glycogen and fats. This time period is termed oxidative or aerobic.

It is important to keep these time periods in mind for conditioning purposes. Specificity of exercise demands that training be very specific to the activity. For example, Mark Spitz won all of his gold medals in the 1972 Olympics in events that fell into the time period from 30 seconds to 2 minutes. That is, all of his events depended upon the optimal training for use of the nonoxidative energy sources. A sprinter should train so as to stress the immediate and nonoxidative energy sources (time periods I and II), while a distance performer would train so as to stress the oxidative energy sources (time period VI). Training for team sports such as soccer and basketball or games like tennis and handball should stress activities that require both nonoxidative and oxidative energy sources (periods III, IV, and V).

This statement should allow the student to better understand the nature of physical exercise and the energy systems involved in the various types of exercises.

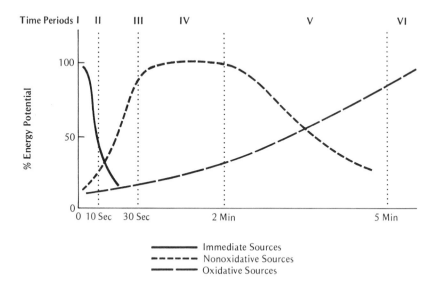

Figure 4–5. Sequence of the activation of energy sources within an active muscle. This figure shows that the energy for a specific exercise arises from different energy sources as a function of the duration of the exercise.

Procedure 1. In small groups the students should list as many favorite activities as possible and locate these in the appropriate time classification.

Teaching Methods *Performance Objective*

The student should be able to categorize activities according to time and energy potential.

Teaching Hint

Have the students organize into small groups. The instructor should suggest different physical activities and the students should estimate the primary energy sources for those activities.

Discussion 1. Develop a list of the activities and the types of training methods that are most appropriate.

Activity	*Time Classification*	*Type of Training*
1. Basketball	Transition V	Primarily short-term and some long-term
2. _____		
3. _____		
4. _____		
5. _____		

2. In the above list, what energy sources are being stressed?
3. Can one simultaneously become a world class athlete in all the classifications?

statement 4

> A Relative Fitness Profile of physical fitness and motor ability criteria aids in developing and maintaining a method of self-evaluation.

Introduction The concept of physical fitness is now as American as the flag, Mom, and apple pie. Presidential commissions and councils are formed, medical groups mobilize, institution such as schools, colleges, and YMCAs get involved. Despite this attention, most Americans fail to recognize the benefits of regular exercise.

Physical fitness is beyond definition, although many have attempted to put it into words. The President's Council on Physical Fitness and Sports has defined physical fitness as "the ability to carry out daily tasks with vigor and alertness, without undue fatigue, and with ample energy to enjoy leisure-time pursuits and to meet unforeseen emergencies."[1] It is proposed that instead of defining physical fitness, a description would be more realistic; one of the best is presented by Johnson and Stolberg:[2]

Health and Fitness Criteria	*Motor Performance Criteria*
Cardiorespiratory capacity	Coordination
Flexibility	Agility
Muscular Endurance	Power
Muscular Strength	Balance
Body Composition	Reaction Time
	Speed

Most of the statements in this book are devoted to the description, assessment, definition, and improvement of these criteria. The Relative Fitness Profile (see Table 4–3, p. 39) has been established to aid students in recognizing where they are, where they must go, and how to get there.

Upon the completion of each task, as they are described in the

[1]*Physical Fitness Research Digest*, H. Harrison Clarke, ed. Washington, D.C.: The Presidents' Council on Physical Fitness and Sports.

[2]Perry Johnson and Donald Stolberg, *Conditioning* (Englewood Cliffs, N.J.: Prentice-Hall, Inc., 1971).

TABLE 4–3. The Relative Fitness Profile

	SOMATOLOGY			
	Statement Reference	*Date*	*Date*	*Date*
Height	5	_____	_____	_____
Weight	5	_____	_____	_____
% of Body Fat	5	_____	_____	_____
Pounds Overweight	6	_____	_____	_____
Somatotype	5	_____	_____	_____
Total Skinfold (4 sites)	5	_____	_____	_____
Girths: Upper Arm	5	_____	_____	_____
Chest	5	_____	_____	_____
Thigh	5	_____	_____	_____
Waist	5	_____	_____	_____
Postural Deviation	14	_____	_____	_____

	THE NEUROMUSCULAR SYSTEM			
Muscular Strength	16	_____	_____	_____
Muscular Endurance	17	_____	_____	_____
Grip Strength	23	_____	_____	_____
Trunk Flexion	15	_____	_____	_____
Trunk Extension	15	_____	_____	_____
Speed (50-yard dash)	23	_____	_____	_____
Agility	23	_____	_____	_____
Reaction Time	23	_____	_____	_____
Balance	23	_____	_____	_____
Power	23	_____	_____	_____
Strength to Arm-Girth Ratio	16	_____	_____	_____

Table 4–3.   Continued

ENERGY SYSTEMS				
Astrand's Bicycle Test	30	_____	_____	_____
Cooper's 12-min Test (Category)	33	_____	_____	_____
Cooper's 1.5-mi Test (Category)	33	_____	_____	_____
Nonoxidative Power	35	_____	_____	_____

ENERGY SUPPORT SYSTEMS				
Resting Heart Rate	32	_____	_____	_____
Harvard Step Test	37	_____	_____	_____
Work Capacity (YMCA Adaptation)	40	_____	_____	_____
Vital Capacity	36	_____	_____	_____
Forced Expiratory Volume (Predicted)	36	_____	_____	_____
Blood Pressure	49	_____	_____	_____
Threshold Heart Rate	41	_____	_____	_____
Cardiac Risk Index	50	_____	_____	_____

statements, the student should record the results in the space provided on the Relative Fitness Profile. The student will then be able to make decisions regarding physical fitness and health. What criteria are important? Can they be measured easily or do they need some sophisticated equipment? Does the student need to improve the individual profile or is a maintenance program suggested?

Procedure   Have the student complete this profile upon the conclusion of each assessment technique. Three columns have been provided for additional testing dates of all or some selected criteria.

Teaching Methods   *Performance Objective*
    The student should be able to record in an organized fashion the performance on each selected test and to use this record for an evaluation of any subsequent retesting.

Teaching Hint
    Stress the importance of periodic assessment. These should be individual to the student. If all the statements in this text are utilized, a relatively comprehensive profile can be established.

Discussion 1. Ask students to list four tests that are the most relevant to their interests.
2. Of those tests listed, what type of program can best meet the students' fitness objectives?

Materials 1. Each statement describes the materials and equipment necessary.
2. The profile may be duplicated and either given to each student or kept in a class file.

chapter 5

Somatology

statement 5

The human body can be classified (somatotyped) according to selected body characteristics.

Introduction Thirty minutes of "people watching" in any large store or on a city street makes clear the wide range of body types.

In 1951 William Sheldon, M.D., devised a series of characteristics designed to classify human body types.[1] These basic body types were termed endomorphic (fat), mesomorphic (muscular), and ectomorphic (skinny). Everyone has some of the characteristics of each body type; thus Sheldon labeled the body types as a three-number series on a scale from 1 to 7. For example, a perfect endomorph would have a rating of 7–1–1, while a true mesomorph a 1–7–1, and a true ectomorph a 1–1–7. The characteristics of each basic type are related to bone structure, muscle mass, fat content, height, weight, and other general characteristics.

Although many factors influence the size, shape, and structure of the human body, heredity plays a crucial role in determining the basic somatotype. Although it is possible to alter the body characteristics, the basic body type remains relatively constant throughout life. When a student assesses his or her basic body type, he or she can gain an understanding of himself or herself and be able to anticipate some of his or her future needs.

In this statement the student shall determine basic somatotype by the Heath-Carter method.[2]

Procedure 1. To determine the *endomorphic* component, the following four skinfold measurements must be taken:

Site	Measurement (mm)
Triceps	_____

[1]See William H. Sheldon, S. S. Stevens, and W. B. Tucker, *Varieties of Human Physique* (New York: Harper & Row, 1951).

[2]B. H. Heath, and J. E. L. Carter, "A Modified Somatotype Method." *American Journal of Physical Anthropology*, 27:57–74, 1967.

Subscapular ______________

Abdominal ______________

Calf ______________

Total ______________

The sum of the three measurements is to be applied to the endomorphic channel in Figure 5–1. Follow the level appropriate for the sum of the three skinfold measures that apply, and note the number at the bottom of the column. This number (1 to 7) is the estimated endomorphic component.

2. The determination of the *mesomorphic* component is difficult when utilizing this particular technique. For the purposes of this lesson the instructor and the student may estimate this component. More

HEATH-CARTER SOMATOTYPE RATING FORM

NAME .... AGE .... SEX: M F NO: ....

OCCUPATION .... ETHNIC GROUP .... DATE ....

PROJECT: .... MEASURED BY: ....

Skinfolds (mm):
Triceps = 10.95
Subcapular = 11.25
Supraliac = 14.30
TOTAL SKINFOLDS = 36.5
Calf = 5.5

TOTAL SKINFOLDS (mm)

Upper Limit	10.9	14.9	18.9	22.9	26.9	31.2	35.8	40.7	46.2	52.2	58.7	65.7	73.2	81.2	89.7	98.9	108.9	119.7	131.2	143.7	157.2	171.9	187.9	204.0
Mid-point	9.0	13.0	17.0	21.0	25.0	29.0	33.5	38.0	43.5	49.0	55.5	62.0	69.5	77.0	85.5	94.0	104.0	114.0	125.5	137.0	150.5	164.0	180.0	196.0
Lower Limit	7.0	11.0	15.0	19.0	23.0	27.0	31.3	(35.9)	40.8	46.3	52.3	58.8	65.8	73.3	81.3	89.8	99.0	109.0	119.8	131.3	143.8	157.3	172.0	188.0
FIRST COMPONENT	½	1	1½	2	2½	3	3½	(4)	4½	5	5½	6	6½	7	7½	8	8½	9	9½	10	10½	11	11½	12

Height (in.) = ☐	55.0	56.5	58.0	59.5	61.0	62.5	64.0	65.5	67.0	68.5	70.0	71.5 ↓	73.0	74.5	76.0	77.5	79.0	80.5	82.0	83.5	85.0	86.5	88.0	89.5
Bone: Humerus (cm) = ☐	5.19	5.34	5.49	5.64	5.78	5.93	6.07	6.22	6.37	6.51	6.65	6.80	6.95	(7.09)	7.24	7.38	7.53	7.67	7.82	7.97	8.11	8.25	8.40	8.55
Femur = ☐	7.41	7.62	7.83	8.04	8.24	8.45	8.66	8.87	9.08	(9.28)	9.49	9.70	9.91	10.12*	10.33	10.53	10.74	10.95	11.16	11.37	11.58	11.79	12.00	12.21
Muscle: Biceps (cm) - (triceps skinfold) = ☐	23.7	24.4	25.0	25.7	26.3	27.0	27.7	28.3	29.0	29.7	30.3	31.0	31.6	32.2	33.0	33.6	34.3	35.0	(35.6)	36.3	37.1	37.8	38.5	39.3
Calf - (calf skinfold) = ☐	27.7	28.5	29.3	30.1	30.8	31.6	32.4	33.2	33.9	34.7	35.5	36.3	37.1	37.8	38.6	(39.4)	40.2	41.0	41.8	42.6	43.4	44.2	45.0	45.8

SECOND COMPONENT: ½ 1 1½ 2 2½ 3 3½ 4 4½ 5 (5½) 6 6½ 7 7½ 8 8½ 9

Weight (lb.) = 191
Ht. / $\sqrt[3]{Wt.}$ = ☐
72 inch.

Upper limit	11.99	12.32	12.53	12.74	12.95	13.15	13.36	13.56	13.77	13.98	14.19	14.39	14.59	14.80	15.01	15.22	15.42	15.63
Mid-point	and	12.16	(12.43)	12.64	12.85	13.05	13.26	13.46	13.67	13.88	14.01	14.29	14.50	14.70	14.91	15.12	15.33	15.53
Lower limit	below	12.00	12.33	12.54	12.75	12.96	13.16	13.37	13.56	13.78	13.99	14.20	14.40	14.60	14.81	15.02	15.23	15.43
THIRD COMPONENT	½	1	(1½)	2	2½	3	3½	4	4½	5	5½	6	6½	7	7½	8	8½	9

	FIRST COMPONENT	SECOND COMPONENT	THIRD COMPONENT	
Anthropometric Somatotype	4	5½	1½	BY: ....
Anthropometric plus Photoscopic Somatotype				RATER: ....

Figure 5–1. The Heath-Carter Somatotype Rating Form. From B.H. Heath and J.E.L. Carter. A Modified Somatotype Method. *American Journal of Physical Anthropology* 27 (1967) 57–74.

appropriate would be to obtain the following measurement. Refer to Teaching Hint 4 to see an example using the measurements.

	Diameters			*Circumferences*	
Humerus	_____	cm	Biceps	_____	cm
Femur	_____	cm	Calf	_____	cm

Note: Both circumferences must be corrected for fat by subtracting the triceps and calf skinfold measures. Skinfolds are measured in mm. To change to cm move the decimal one place to the left prior to subtraction.

3. To determine the *ectomorphic* component, apply the student's height and weight to the nomogram (Figure 5–2). The figure obtained from the center column is used to locate the ectomorphic component (Figure 5–1) by reading across the *Ectomorphy* row to the appropriate figure.

Teaching Methods

Performance Objective

The student should be able to estimate individual somatotypes utilizing the charts and techniques described.

Teaching Hints

1. The teacher should discuss each body type. A presentation with pictures of famous people from magazines is effective. The references at the end of this section, as well as those in the footnotes, provide a reading background for somatotyping.
2. Students in small groups could evaluate each other instead of using the measurement method. However, the instructor must spend much more time explaining the observational techniques of somatotyping.
3. Posters, mobiles, bulletin boards, comic strip characters, etc. can be used effectively in this lesson.
4. A example of how to use this procedure:

   An 18 year-old student is 6 feet tall, weighs 191 pounds, and has skinfold measures totaling 36.5. Reading along the first component row (endomorphic) of Figure 5–1 we find, after locating 35.9 and reading downward, an endomorphic component of 4.

   Using Figure 5–2 for determining the cube root of height divided into weight we discover a figure of 12.45. Reading along the third component row (ectomorphic) and reading down the column, we find an ectomorphic component of 1½.

   The mesomorphic component is more difficult to determine. With a knowledge of the first and third components it is possible for the instructor and the student to estimate the mesomorphic component.

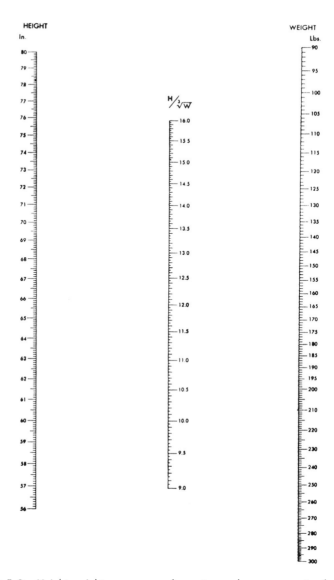

Figure 5-2. Height-weight nomogram for ectomorphy component of somato-typing. By permission of William Sheldon. *Atlas of Men* New York Harper and Row, 1954.

For those wishing a more precise determination the following description will serve as a guide. The compartment at the left of the rating form (Figure 5-1) contains five boxes in which the measurements described should be placed. In this example: Height = 72, Humerus = 7.1, Femur = 9.2 Biceps (corrected for fat) = 35.4 and the calf (corrected for fat) = 39. 6. The correction for skinfold of the biceps and calf circumferences is done by subtracting the biceps and calf skinfolds. It must be noted that skinfold measurements are generally recorded in

47

millimeters (mm) whereas circumferences are recorded in centimeters (cm). To change mm to cm simply move the decimal one place to the left. In the example illustrated the calf skinfold of 7.1 mm would become .7cm and the tricep skinfold of 11.0 mm is corrected to 1.1 cm. Each box is opposite a row which contains corresponding numbers. An arrow facing downward should be placed at the number corresponding to the actual height. In this case, the arrow will be placed at 71.5 which is closer to 72, the actual height, than the next number along the row 73. Each row should then be circled at the appropriate number corresponding to the listed measure (humerus = 7.09, femur = 9.28, biceps = 35.6, and calf = 39.4.) Next, starting at the circled measure most proximate to the left hand margin (e.g., femur = 9.28) count the number of displacements to the right of each circled number. That is, humerus = 4, Biceps = 9, and calf = 6 for a total of 19. Divide the displacements (19) by 4 which equals 4.75. Now count 4.75 places from the measure closest to the left hand margin (femur) and place an asterisk at that point. Drop a line from the height column to the femur and asterisk row. Count over from the height marker to the asterisk.

A displacement of 2.75 to the right is noted. Locate 4 in the second component row, and move 2.75 places to the right. For this student, 5½ would be circled.

Our demonstration student would have a present somatotype of 4–5½–1½ as determined by the Heath-Carter Method.

Knowledge of somatotype has many other uses for proper health and fitness planning. The student can identify weight gain with age, guide future activity selection, and uncover health risks related to body type.

5. The teacher can find a careful description of the exact locations for obtaining skinfolds, circumferences, and diameters as presented by Behnke and Wilmore.[3]

Discussion
1. Can basic somatotypes be altered?
2. Can slight alterations in some of the components of each somatotype be made by appropriate exercises, diets, etc.?
3. Circle your feelings about your body type:
   A. I dislike my body intensely.
   B. I dislike my body type, but intend to slightly alter it however possible.
   C. I am stuck with a body and must make the best of it.
   D. My body is O.K. I hope to maintain it just like it is.
4. What role does heredity play in determining somatotype?

[3]Albert R. Behnke and Jack H. Wilmore, *Evaluation and Regulation of Body Build and Composition.* Englewood Cliffs, N.J.: Prentice-Hall, Inc., 1974. Chap. 3.

Materials   1. All charts and nomograms are provided.

2. Lange skinfold calipers, wooden anthiopometric calipers, and cloth tape measure. These may be purchased from the J. A. Preston Corp., 71 Fifth Ave., New York, N.Y. 10003.

statement 6

The composition of the body can be estimated to determine the amount of body fat.

Introduction According to some authorities, obesity is of epidemic proportions in the U.S. An abundance of food and our high standard of living is partially responsible for the creation of this problem. Consequently, people should develop an intelligent approach to the normalization of body weight. One such approach involves the determination of a proper body weight for a given height and body build through the assessment of body fat. An examination of the frequently used height and weight charts reveals the inadequacies in estimating body weight from the given height and body classifications. A superior method would appear to result from an assessment of body fat. This component is measured in the laboratory biochemically using radioactive potassium or by underwater weighing. Both these methods, however, involve sophisticated measurement techniques and are impractical for utilization in the schools. Several modified techniques are available which can be applied to large groups requiring only very simple equipment. Each method must be applied only to the population from which it was derived. We are suggesting Parizkova's[1] nomogram for boys and girls age 9 to 16 and Sloan and de V. Weir's[2] nomogram for the population 17 to 26.

Body fat may be defined as the amount of total body weight that is fatty tissue and is usually expressed in terms of a percentage of actual body weight. A study of the literature shows body-fat standards for Americans to range from 12 to 19 percent for males and 20 to 25 percent for females.

For this lesson we will use 16 percent for males and 23 percent for females as the upper "normal" limit of body fat. With this information, we can now determine the number of pounds over or under

[1]J. Parizkova, "Total Body Fat and Skinfold Thickness on Children," *Metabolism*, 10 (1961), 794–807.

[2]A. W. Sloan and J. B. de V. Weir, "Nomograms for prediction of body density and total body fat from skinfold measurements." *Journal Applied Physiology* (1970), 221–22.

the recommended amount of fat and we should be able to more precisely calculate the "ideal" body weight for a given height and body build.

Procedure   1. Skinfold measures should be obtained and recorded for the population and method to be used.

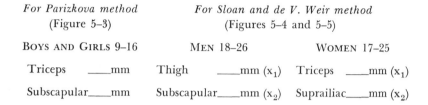

For Parizkova method
(Figure 5–3)

BOYS AND GIRLS 9–16

Triceps   ____mm

Subscapular____mm

For Sloan and de V. Weir method
(Figures 5–4 and 5–5)

MEN 18–26

Thigh   ____mm (x_1)

Subscapular____mm (x_2)

WOMEN 17–25

Triceps   ____mm (x_1)

Suprailiac____mm (x_2)

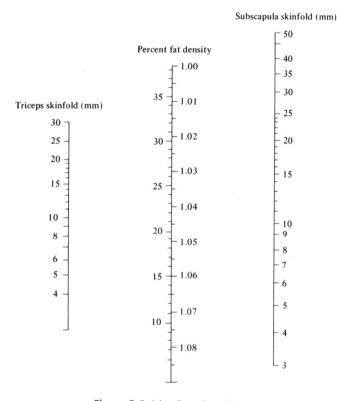

Figure 5–3 (a). Boys 9 to 12.

Figure 5–3 (a–d). Parizkova nomograms for body fat prediction based on triceps and subscapular skinfold measurements. By permission of J. Parizkova, "Total body fat and skinfold thickness in children," *Metabolism* 10 (1961), 794–807.

2. The appropriate nomogram is read by placing a straightedged object or string on the measured skinfold thickness. The intersection with the middle column gives the figure for percent fat.

3. To determine pounds over or under recommended fat amount, use the following formula:

$$\text{Pounds Over/Under in Fat} = \text{Actual Body Weight} \times \\ (\text{Body Fat \%} - 16\% \text{ or } 23\%)$$

(In the formula 16% should be used by men and 23% by women.)

Teaching Methods

Performance Objectives

1. The student should be able to determine the percentage of body fat based on the appropriate nomograms.
2. Calculate the pounds over or under the recommended amount of fat using the given formula.

Teaching Hints

1. This statement integrates nicely with Statement 5. Three of the four skinfold measurements utilized in this statement were needed for somatotyping.

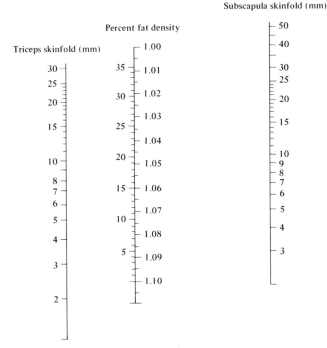

Figure 5–3 (b). Boys 13 to 16.

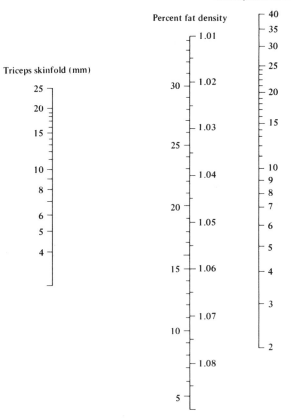

Figure 5–3 (c). Girls 9 to 12.

2. Use 16 percent for men and 23 percent for women as the upper limits for body fat percentage when calculating pounds over fat. These percentages are only guidelines and some students may decide upon a percent of body fat lower than these upper limits as a goal. For example, a young man may decide on 10 percent body fat instead of 16 percent as an upper limit.

3. An example of calculating pounds over or under the recommended amount of fat:

A 165-pound male has a body-fat percentage of 21. Using the formula given in Procedure 3, apply the given information.

$$\text{Pounds over/under in fat} = 165 \, (.21 - .16)$$

$$= 165 \, (.05)$$

$$= 8.25 \text{ lbs}$$

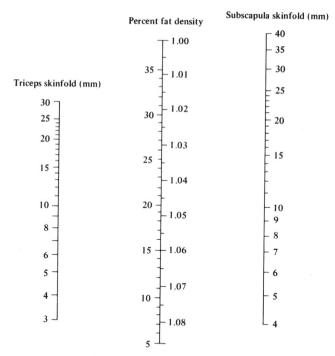

Figure 5–3 (d). Girls 13 to 16.

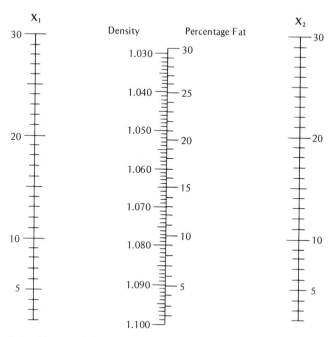

Figure 5–4. Sloan and de V. Weir nomogram for body fat prediction in men based on thigh (X₁) and subscapular (X₂) skinfold measurements. By permission of A. W. Sloan and J. B. deV.Weir, "Nomogram for prediction of body density and total body fat from skinfold measurements," *Journal of Applied Physiology* 28 (1970) 221–222.

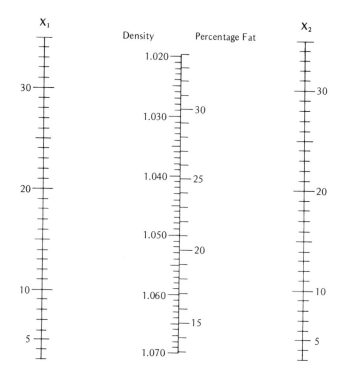

Figure 5–5. Sloan and de V. Weir nomogram for body fat prediction in women based on thigh (X₁) and subscapular (X₂) skinfold measurements. By permission of A.W. Sloan and J.B. de V. Weir. "Nomogram for prediction of body density and total body fat from skinfold measurements." *Journal Applied Physiology.* 28 (1970) 221–222.

This person is then considered 8.25 pounds above the desired 16 percent of body fat. With this information, the student can more accurately plan for future weight control.

4. For athletes, the discussion might involve two recent studies revealing that male members of the U.S. Nordic Ski Team showed an average percent of body fat of 8.5, while another study cites 15 percent body fat for collegiate women gymnasts.

5. Several other methods are available for determining body fat percentage; for example, the YMCA has recently published a method that has possibility for use in the schools.[3]

Discussion   1. Discuss some of the health conditions which obesity and overweight may cause a predisposition to, such as diabetes, high blood pressure, pulmonary congestion, heart disease, etc.

[3]Clayton Myers, Lawrence Golding, and Wayne Sinning, *The Y's Way to Fitness* (Emmaus, Pa.: Rodale Press, 1973).

2. Calculate the pounds necessary to achieve an ideal goal involving a lesser body fat percentage. For example, use a 10 percent goal for men and 18 percent for women.
3. What weight does each student consider appropriate for his or her height and body build based on these calculations?
4. This information should be placed on the Relative Fitness Profile for later comparison. For example, it would be meaningful for the students to examine this percent of body fat several times during the year. Also, fitness categories based on some way of the cardio-vascular testing and body-fat percentage would prove interesting. Statement 9 could use the 12-minute or 1.5-mile run information instead of estimating physical activity.

Materials   Lange skinfold calipers. (Source is listed in Statement 5.) If these calipers cannot be purchased, a mm ruler and scientific calipers can be used. These probably could be borrowed from the science department.

statement 7

There is a difference between being overweight and being obese.

Introduction
According to Jean Mayer, a difference exists between being overweight and being obese.[1] To be overweight is simply to be above the charts in weight in relation to height, while obesity may be defined as having a percentage of body fat above 39 percent.

To do this lesson, the students should already have determined body-fat percentage. Any student with 39 percent body fat or above would be considered obese. Another method for determining obesity has been established by Seltzer and Mayer based on the thickness of the triceps skinfold.[2]

To determine "overweightness," the student will need to match height, weight, and frame size on Tables 5-1 and 5-2. A weight beyond the value given there for a given height and frame size would place a person in the overweight category.

Procedure
1. "Overweightness" is determined by locating the student's ideal weight based on height and frame size from Tables 5–1 and 5–2. Did the students have difficulty determining frame size? Are any students above the upper limit in terms of body-fat percent, but below the 39 percent figure? If so, this would indicate overweightness, but not obesity.
2. "Obesity" may be evaluated by utilizing the triceps skinfold measurement using Table 5–3. Is this in harmony with the students' finding regarding body-fat percentage and the 39 percent figure?

Teaching Methods
Performance Objectives
1. The student should learn to determine individual overweight and obesity levels.

[1] J. Mayer, *Overweight* (Englewood Cliffs, N.J.: Prentice-Hall, Inc., 1968).
[2] C. C. Seltzer and Jean Mayer, "A Simple Criterion of Obesity," *Postgraduate Medicine*, 38, no. 2 (1965), A-101.

TABLE 5–1.   New Desirable Weights for Women.

Height (with shoes, 2-inch heels)	Small Frame	Medium Frame	Large Frame
4′ 10″	92–98	96–107	104–119
4′ 11″	94–101	98–110	106–122
5′ 0″	96–104	101–113	109–125
1″	99–107	104–116	112–128
2″	102–110	107–119	115–131
3″	105–113	110–122	118–134
4″	108–116	113–126	121–138
5″	111–119	116–130	125–142
6″	114–123	120–135	129–146
7″	118–127	124–139	133–150
8″	122–131	128–143	137–154
9″	126–135	132–147	141–158
10″	130–140	136–151	145–163
11″	134–144	140–155	149–168
6′ 0″	138–148	144–159	153–173

By permission of Metropolitan Life Insurance Company.

TABLE 5–2.   New Desirable Weights for Men.

Height (with shoes, 1-inch heels)	Small Frame	Medium Frame	Large Frame
5′ 2″	112–120	118–129	126–141
3″	115–123	121–133	129–144
4″	118–126	124–136	142–148
5″	121–129	127–139	135–152
6″	124–133	130–143	138–156
7″	128–137	134–147	142–161
8″	132–141	138–152	147–166
9″	136–145	142–156	151–170
10″	140–150	146–160	155–174
11″	144–154	150–165	159–179
6′ 0″	148–158	154–170	164–184
1″	152–162	158–175	168–189
2″	156–167	162–180	173–194
3″	160–171	167–185	178–199
4″	164–175	172–190	182–204

By permission of Metropolitan Life Insurance Company.

TABLE 5–3. Obesity Standards in Caucasian Americans.

	Minimum Triceps Skinfold Thickness Indicating Obesity (Millimeters)				
Age (years)	Males	Females	Age (years)	Males	Females
5	12	14	18	15	27
6	12	15	19	15	27
7	13	16	20	16	28
8	14	17	21	17	28
9	15	18	22	18	28
10	16	20	23	18	28
11	17	21	24	19	28
12	18	22	25	20	29
13	18	23	26	20	29
14	17	23	27	21	29
15	16	24	28	22	29
16	15	25	29	22	29
17	14	26	30–50	23	30

Source: C. C. Seltzer, and J. Mayer, "A Simple Criterion of Obesity," *Postgraduate Medicine*, 38, no. 2 (1965), A-101.

2. The student should also be able to list two criticisms of using the height and weight charts for determining "normal" weight.

Teaching Hints
1. This statement integrates very nicely with Statements 5 and 6 because the triceps skinfold will have been obtained for these statements.
2. It might be interesting to determine the percentage of the class that is overweight or obese.

Discussion
1. List two criticisms of the Life Insurance Company's height and weight charts.
2. Mayer says that 16 percent of all teenagers are obese. Does this percentage agree with that of your class?
3. Define the terms "overweight" and "obese." What is meant by saying a person has over/under the recommended amount of fat?
4. Match the following:

_____ A. Overweight

1. a body fat percentage above 39.

_____ B. A high percentage of fat

2. a weight above the charts relative to height.

_____ C. A low percentage of fat

3. above the norms for body fat but below the obese level.

_____ D. Obese

4. below the norms for body fat.

Materials
1. Lange skinfold calipers as previously described.
2. Metropolitan Life Insurance Company charts and Seltzer and Mayer's "Obesity Standard" table.

statement 8

The lifetime pattern for the gain in body weight is related to individual somatotypes.

Introduction It is clear that as a person grows older there is an increase in body weight and the amount of body fat and a decrease in the amount of muscle.[1] Experimental evidence indicates that there is a pattern of weight gain for each somatotype. Knowledge of the expected weight-gain patterns can be used as a guide to properly plan for future weight-control problems. This knowledge will indicate the diet and exercise modifications necessary for achievement of these goals.

Procedure 1. The students should be somatotyped as shown in Statement 5.
2. Table 5–4 gives the expected weight gain with age. Find the somato-type heading, read down the lefthand column to the correct height, and read across for the predicted body weight at each of the three ages listed for the appropriate height.

Teaching Methods *Performance Objectives*

The student should be able to determine the individual weight-gain pattern at ages 18, 38, and 63 based on Sheldon's statistics.

Teaching Hints

Exact somatotyping is impossible. Nevertheless, a general trend in weight gain can be predicted. A high school junior may be somato-typed as a 5-4-3, but because of the range in error for this method, this student may be 5-4-2, 4-5-2, or 4-5-3. The important point of the lesson, however, is that this range of somatotype will show a weight gain over the years of 40 to 50 pounds. Consequently, the important factor of this lesson is not the identification of somatotype, but the pattern of weight increase.

[1] Lawrence B. Oscai. "The Role of Exercise in Weight Control," *Exercise and Sport Sciences Reviews* (Jack H. Wilmore, ed.). New York: Academic Press, pp. 103–125, 1973.

TABLE 5–4.   Weight Gain with Age for various Body Types.

	721			731			621			631		
		Age			Age			Age			Age	
Height	18	38	63	18	38	63	18	38	63	18	38	63
75	292	427	. .	310	465	. .	233	284	. .	245	298	311
74	281	409	. .	298	447	. .	223	272	. .	234	286	298
73	270	393	. .	286	429	. .	215	261	. .	225	274	286
72	259	377	. .	274	412	. .	207	251	. .	216	264	275
71	248	361	. .	263	395	. .	198	241	. .	207	253	263
70	238	346	. .	252	378	. .	190	231	. .	199	243	253
69	228	331	. .	241	363	. .	182	222	. .	191	234	242
68	218	317	. .	231	347	. .	174	212	. .	183	224	233
67	208	304	. .	221	332	. .	167	203	. .	175	214	222
66	199	289	. .	211	317	. .	159	194	. .	167	204	211
65	190	278	. .	202	303	. .	152	185	. .	159	195	203
64	182	264	. .	193	290	. .	145	176	. .	152	186	193
63	173	253	. .	184	276	. .	138	168	. .	145	177	184
62	165	240	. .	175	263	. .	132	160	. .	138	169	176
61	157	230	. .	167	251	. .	125	153	. .	131	161	168

By permission of William Sheldon, *Atlas of Men*. New York: Harper & Row, 1954.

	162			163			262			154		
		Age			Age			Age			Age	
Height	18	38	63	18	38	63	18	38	63	18	38	63
75	196	204	207	187	191	195	202	231	236	171	175	178
74	188	195	200	179	184	187	194	222	227	163	167	171
73	181	187	191	172	177	180	186	212	218	156	160	164
72	173	180	183	165	169	173	179	204	209	150	154	157
71	166	173	175	158	163	166	172	196	201	144	148	151
70	159	166	168	152	156	159	165	188	193	138	142	145
69	153	159	161	145	150	152	157	179	184	133	136	139
68	146	142	154	139	144	145	151	171	176	127	130	133
67	139	146	148	133	137	139	144	164	168	121	124	127
66	133	139	141	127	131	133	137	156	161	116	119	121
65	127	133	135	122	125	127	131	149	154	111	113	116
64	121	127	128	116	119	121	125	142	146	106	108	110
63	116	121	122	110	114	116	119	136	139	101	103	105
62	110	115	116	105	108	110	114	130	133	96	99	100
61	105	110	111	100	103	105	108	123	127	92	94	96

TABLE 5–4   (Continued)

Height	253			254			354		
	Age			Age			Age		
	18	38	63	18	38	63	18	38	63
75	183	201	210	177	192	199	186	213	221
74	176	193	201	170	184	191	178	205	212
73	169	185	193	163	177	184	170	196	203
72	162	177	185	156	169	176	164	188	195
71	156	170	177	150	163	169	157	181	187
70	149	163	170	144	156	162	151	173	180
69	143	157	164	138	150	156	145	166	172
68	137	150	156	132	143	149	139	159	165
67	131	143	149	126	137	142	132	152	158
66	125	137	143	120	131	136	126	145	151
65	119	131	136	115	125	130	121	138	144
64	114	125	130	110	119	124	115	132	137
63	109	119	124	105	114	118	110	126	131
62	104	113	119	100	108	113	105	120	124
61	99	108	113	95	103	107	100	114	119

Height	641			642			651			532		
	Age			Age			Age			Age		
	18	38	63	18	38	63	18	38	63	18	38	63
75	262	339	. .	248	318	324	282	373		206	253	258
74	251	326	. .	238	307	311	270	359	. .	198	243	248
73	241	313	. .	229	294	299	260	345	. .	189	232	237
72	232	300	. .	220	282	287	249	331	. .	182	223	227
71	223	287	. .	221	270	275	238	316	. .	174	214	219
70	214	275	. .	203	260	264	229	302	. .	167	206	210
69	204	264	. .	193	249	253	219	289	. .	161	197	202
68	196	253	. .	186	238	242	209	277	. .	154	189	193
67	187	341	. .	178	228	231	200	264	. .	147	180	184
66	179	231	. .	169	217	221	191	253	. .	140	172	176
65	171	220	. .	162	208	211	183	241	. .	134	164	168
64	163	210	. .	154	198	202	174	231	. .	128	157	160
63	156	201	. .	147	189	192	167	220	. .	122	149	153
62	148	191	. .	141	180	183	159	210	. .	116	142	146
61	141	182	. .	134	172	175	152	200	. .	111	135	139

TABLE 5–4 (Continued)

Height	541			542			543		
	Age			Age			Age		
	18	38	63	18	38	63	18	38	63
75	229	286	299	217	269	280	206	255	259
74	221	275	287	208	259	269	198	245	249
73	211	263	274	199	248	257	190	235	239
72	203	253	263	191	238	247	183	226	230
71	195	243	252	184	229	237	176	217	221
70	187	233	242	177	219	227	168	208	212
69	179	224	232	169	210	218	161	200	203
68	171	214	222	162	201	209	154	191	194
67	164	205	212	155	192	200	147	182	186
66	156	196	202	148	183	191	140	174	177
65	149	187	193	141	175	182	134	166	169
64	142	178	184	134	167	174	128	159	162
63	136	170	176	128	159	166	122	151	154
62	130	162	168	122	152	158	117	144	147
61	123	155	160	116	145	151	111	137	140

Height	344			434			443			444		
	Age			Age			Age			Age		
	18	38	63	18	38	63	18	38	63	18	38	63
75	175	196	205	178	201	210	189	223	234	183	212	221
74	168	189	197	170	193	201	181	214	224	176	204	212
73	162	181	189	164	185	193	174	206	216	169	196	204
72	155	173	181	157	177	185	167	197	207	163	189	196
71	148	167	174	151	170	178	160	189	198	155	180	187
70	142	160	167	145	163	170	154	182	190	149	173	180
69	137	153	160	139	157	164	147	174	183	143	166	172
68	131	147	153	133	150	157	141	167	175	137	159	165
67	125	140	146	127	143	150	135	159	167	131	152	158
66	119	134	140	121	137	143	129	152	160	125	145	151
65	114	128	133	116	131	136	123	145	152	119	138	144
64	109	122	127	110	125	130	117	138	145	114	132	137
63	104	116	121	105	119	124	112	132	139	109	126	131
62	99	111	116	100	113	118	106	126	132	103	120	124
61	94	105	110	96	108	113	101	120	126	99	114	119

TABLE 5–4   (Continued)

	271			371			261			361		
		Age			Age			Age			Age	
Height	18	38	63	18	38	63	18	38	63	18	38	63
75	228	266	271	238	292	. .	212	241	249	221	253	277
74	219	255	260	229	280	. .	203	232	239	211	252	266
73	211	245	249	220	269	. .	195	222	230	203	242	255
72	202	236	240	212	259	. .	188	214	221	195	233	245
71	194	226	230	203	249	. .	180	205	212	187	224	235
70	186	217	220	195	238	. .	173	196	205	180	215	226
69	178	208	211	187	229	. .	166	188	196	172	206	216
68	170	199	202	179	219	. .	159	180	187	165	197	207
67	162	189	192	171	210	. .	152	172	179	158	188	198
66	155	181	184	163	200	. .	145	165	171	151	180	189
65	148	173	175	156	191	. .	138	157	163	144	172	180
64	141	165	167	148	183	. .	132	150	156	137	164	172
63	134	157	159	141	174	. .	126	143	149	131	157	164
62	128	150	152	135	166	. .	120	136	142	124	149	156
61	122	143	145	128	158	. .	114	130	135	119	142	149

	362			461			352			451		
		Age			Age			Age			Age	
Height	18	38	63	18	38	63	18	38	63	18	38	63
75	211	249	260	236	302	. .	200	232	241	214	267	282
74	204	239	249	226	288	. .	191	222	231	205	256	271
73	196	230	239	217	277	. .	184	214	222	197	246	261
72	188	221	230	209	266	. .	177	206	214	190	236	251
71	181	212	221	201	256	. .	170	198	206	181	226	240
70	173	204	212	193	246	. .	162	189	196	174	217	230
69	166	195	203	185	236	. .	156	181	188	167	208	221
68	159	187	194	177	226	. .	149	173	180	160	199	212
67	152	179	186	169	216	. .	142	166	172	153	190	202
66	145	170	177	161	206	. .	136	158	165	146	181	193
65	138	163	169	154	197	. .	130	151	157	139	173	184
64	132	155	162	147	188	. .	124	144	150	133	165	176
63	126	148	154	140	179	. .	118	137	143	127	157	168
62	120	141	147	134	171	. .	113	131	137	121	150	160
61	114	135	140	127	163	. .	107	125	130	115	143	153

TABLE 5–4   (Continued)

Height	452			453		
	Age			Age		
	18	38	63	18	38	63
75	206	251	264	197	236	250
74	198	241	254	189	227	240
73	190	232	244	182	218	230
72	183	223	235	175	210	222
71	175	213	225	167	201	212
70	168	205	216	160	193	204
69	161	196	207	154	185	194
68	154	188	198	147	177	187
67	147	179	188	141	169	178
66	140	171	181	134	161	170
65	134	164	172	128	154	163
64	128	156	165	122	147	155
63	122	149	157	117	140	148
62	117	142	150	111	134	141
61	111	135	143	106	127	133

Height	127			126			136			236		
	Age			Age			Age			Age		
	18	38	63	18	38	63	18	38	63	18	38	63
75	136	138	138	143	146	148	149	152	156	155	162	165
74	130	132	132	137	140	142	143	146	149	149	156	159
73	125	127	127	132	134	136	137	140	143	142	150	153
72	120	122	122	127	129	130	132	134	137	136	143	146
71	116	118	118	122	124	125	127	129	132	131	137	140
70	111	113	113	117	119	120	122	124	126	125	131	135
69	107	108	108	112	114	115	117	119	121	120	126	129
68	102	104	104	107	109	110	112	114	116	115	121	123
67	98	99	99	102	104	105	107	109	111	110	115	118
66	93	95	95	98	100	100	102	104	106	105	110	113
65	89	90	90	94	95	96	97	99	101	100	105	108
64	84	86	86	89	91	91	93	95	97	96	100	103
63	81	82	82	85	87	88	89	90	92	91	96	98
62	77	78	78	81	82	83	85	86	88	87	91	93
61	73	74	74	77	78	79	81	82	84	83	87	89

TABLE 5–4   (Continued)

	145			235			245			345		
		Age			Age			Age			Age	
Height	18	38	63	18	38	63	18	38	63	18	38	63
75	158	161	164	160	168	173	165	176	182	169	186	193
74	151	154	157	153	161	167	158	168	174	162	178	186
73	145	148	151	146	154	160	152	162	168	156	171	179
72	139	142	145	141	148	154	146	156	161	150	165	172
71	134	136	139	135	142	147	140	150	155	143	157	164
70	128	131	133	130	136	141	134	144	149	137	151	158
69	123	125	127	124	131	135	129	138	143	131	145	151
68	118	120	122	119	125	129	123	132	137	126	139	145
67	112	115	116	114	119	123	117	125	129	120	132	138
66	107	109	111	109	114	118	112	119	124	115	126	132
65	102	105	106	104	109	112	107	114	118	109	121	126
64	98	100	101	99	104	107	102	109	113	104	115	120
63	93	95	97	94	99	102	97	104	108	100	110	115
62	89	91	92	90	94	98	93	99	103	92	105	109
61	85	87	88	86	90	93	88	94	98	90	100	104

Discussion   1. Is it necessary to gain weight with age as predicted?

2. List at least three methods that might alter the predicted weight-gain pattern.

Materials   Table 5–4.

statement 9

> **Physical activity affects the composition of the body.**

Introduction Research evidence is available indicating that body fat is lower in physically active people. Parizkova found that during a four-week exercise program, body fat decreased.[1] However, after seven weeks of inactivity the body fat returned to the pre-exercise levels.[1] Several researchers have confirmed the fact that a significant decrease in body fat occurs in active people as opposed to those who are sedentary.

It seems then that we can conclude that with exercise of the proper intensity and duration, it is possible to decrease the percentage of body fat and to increase the percentage of lean body weight.

Procedure 1. The students should categorize themselves according to their normal activity level as follows:

Active:	An athlete in training or a person who exercises at a level comparable to running at least 2 miles a day, 5 days a week.
Moderately Active:	Planned recreation at least 3 days a week or involvement in a heavy occupation such as construction or farming.
Sedentary:	Only normal daily activities such as eating, sleeping, sitting, talking, a sedentary job, or attending school.

2. Knowing the percentage of body fat (Statement 6), each student should insert this information in the appropriate category on the suggested chart drawn on the blackboard.

Body Fat %

Active   _____

Moderately Active   _____

Sedentary   _____

[2]J. Parizkova, "Impact of Age, Diet, and Exercise on Man's Body Composition," *Annals of the New York Academy of Sciences*, 110 (1963), p. 661.

4. Select a student to calculate the average body-fat percent for each activity category.

Teaching Methods

Performance Objective

The student should be able to determine, on the basis of class experimentation, the relationship between physical activity and the amount of body fat.

Teaching Hints

1. The procedure is self-explanatory. The reduction of body fat is an important "training effect." This aspect should be stressed in class discussion. Some students may want to study themselves over the school year.
2. Instead of using the subjective evaluation of activity levels suggested in Procedure 1, a more precise method is to use the results from the bicycle ergometer (Statement 30) or the 12-minute or 1.5 mile (Statement 33) tests.

Discussion

1. Is there a relationship between body-fat percent and physical activity?
2. How do you account for the fact that weight may remain the same but body fat may decrease in some individuals during physical training?

Materials

Same as in Statement 6.

statement **10**

> **There is an increase in the amount of energy needed to exercise when the body is overweight.**

Introduction   Excess weight serves as an extra load when any physical activity is performed. Studies have shown that there is an increase in the amount of energy needed to perform most tasks, whether the type of obesity is spontaneously developed (by overeating) or produced experimentally.

This experiment simulates a 20-pound weight gain in each student. The measurement of heart rate is used to predict energy cost.

Procedure   1. Have the student take a resting heart rate by palpating the carotid artery. This is probably the most efficient location for the taking of an exercise heart rate. Proper instruction in the use of this technique will facilitate ease of obtaining accurate data.

2. The students should then step up and down on a bench, bleachers, stairs, or chair for one minute at a cadence of 30 steps per minute (one step is defined as up with the left foot, up with right foot, down with the left, and down with the right). A metronome set at 120 beats per minute helps in this exercise. Upon the completion of one minute of stepping, the student should immediately take a 10-second pulse count as previously explained. This pulse count, when multiplied by six, will give a reasonable approximation of the exercise heart rate per minute.

3. The student should rest until the heart rate has returned to within five beats of the original resting rate before proceeding to the next section of this experiment.

4. Repeat the step test with a pack loaded with 20 pounds of weights. Take the heartbeat rate (HR) at the completion of the test as previously described.

5. Chart the results

	Resting HR	*Exercise HR*
Normal Body Weight	_____	_____
Experimental Obesity	_____	_____

Teaching Methods

Performance Objective

The students should be able to observe the effects of experimental obesity on the responses of the cardiovascular (CV) system, and indirectly on energy expenditure, related to an exercise task.

Teaching Hint

For best results the students should complete at least two trials of the normal condition and two of the experimental conditions. Mean scores of the two conditions are important for discussion purposes.

Discussion

1. Account for the response of the CV system to the normal weight and to the increased-weight condition.
2. List two possible reasons for maintaining normal body weight.
3. What percent weight gain was the added 20 lbs for each student?

$$\% \text{ Weight Gain} = \frac{20 \text{ lbs}}{\text{Actual Body Weight}} \times 100$$

4. Does exercise in an overweight person require more energy? In terms of weight reduction, can exercise play a significant role in an overweight individual?

Materials

1. Packs.
2. 20 lbs of weights.
3. Metronome.
4 A stepping bench.

statement **11**

Success in sports may have a relationship to somatotype.

Introduction Some evidence is available to suggest that a choice of activities might be considered according to somatotype.[1] For example, as shown in Figure 5–6 when successful athletes are placed in their respective sports on the somachart, there is a distinct grouping for each sport. Football players cluster in the upper lefthand corner, while long-distance runners group to the right of the center axis.

Although people should not be discouraged from participation in any sport, some guidance based on this information might eliminate later discouragement.

Procedure 1. Locate the students' somatotypes on the somatochart.
2. Complete the following table by somatocharting the following sports and placing the number of appropriate area from the somatochart in the righthand column. (For example, cross-country skiers would undoubtedly be in area 5.)

Sport	Somatochart Area
Cross-Country Skiing	_____
Bicycle Racing	_____
Tennis	_____
Sprinting	_____
Swimming	_____
Shot Put and Discus Events	_____
High Jump and Long Jump	_____

[1] J. E. L. Carter, "The Somatotypes of Athletes—A Review." *Human Biology.* 42:536–569, 1970.

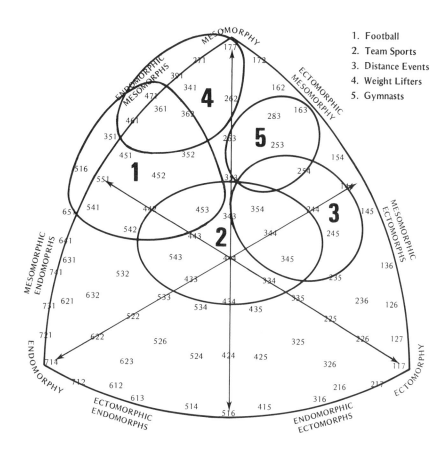

1. Football
2. Team Sports
3. Distance Events
4. Weight Lifters
5. Gymnasts

Figure 5–6. Somatotype distribution of athletes. The average somatotype for various sports is plotted on the above somatochart. This technique does indicate that differences do exist in somatotype among sports. Although no student should be discouraged from participation in any sport it does appear that as higher levels of competition are reached the differences in somatotype patterns do narrow. Adapted from the data of J.E.L. Carter, "The Somatotypes of Athletes—A Review," *Human Biology* 42 (1970), 536–69.

Teaching Methods

Performance Objective

Each student should be able to determine which activities are compatible with his or her body type for future sports success.

Teaching Hints

The students should locate their somatotypes on the somatochart, then answer the questions below.

Discussion   1. The students should list three favorite sports or recreational activities.
2. Are these activities compatible to the students' somatotypes?
3. Should an individual limit sports participation to only those activities which seem to indicate success on the somatochart?
4. Is somatocharting only important for those seeking competition?
5. Which somatotype grouping is most apt to have coronary attacks in adult years?
6. Which somatotype would be most likely to exercise throughout life? Why?

Materials   Somatochart.

statement 12

> Body build may be related to temperament, personality, and achievement needs.

Introduction   William Sheldon not only characterized the physical aspects of man, but because he was a psychologist he also attempted to describe temperament and personality as related to body type.[1]

As is true of the physical somatotype characteristics, the psychological characteristics are scored as a combination of Sheldon's three components. To assess the psychological scores, the student will take the self-description test (Table 5–5) developed by Cortes and Gatti.[2]

Procedure   1. The student should take the Self-Description Test.
2. Count the number of adjectives that the student selected in each of the three categories (Table 5–6). For example if the totals are 10, 6, and 5 the student has predominantly endomorphic traits. A 6, 10, 5 score would be high in the mesomorphic category.
3. Does the personality score relate to the primary physical components identified in Statement 5?

Teaching Methods   *Performance Objective*

The student should be able to identify predominant temperament traits by taking the Cortes and Gatti test and then determine how they relate to his or her body build.

Discussion   1. List several ways in which a knowledge of physique and temperament could help in better self-understanding.
2. Do you think temperament and physique are related?

Materials   Cortes and Gatti's Self-Description Test and Key.

[1] William Sheldon, S. S. Stevens, and W. B. Tucker, *Varieties of Human Physique* (New York: Harper and Row), 1951.
[2] J. B. Cortes and F. M. Gatti, "Physique and Propensity," *Psychology Today* 4 (1970), p. 42–44.

TABLE 5–5. Self-Description Test.

Below are some statements for you to complete about yourself. Fill in each blank with a word from the suggested list following each statement. For any blank, three in each statement, you may select any word from the list of twelve immediately below. An exact word to fit you may not be in the list, but select the words that seem to fit most closely with the way you are:

1. I feel most of the time _____, _____, and _____.

calm	relaxed	complacement
anxious	confident	reticent
cheerful	tense	energetic
contented	impetuous	self-conscious

2. When I study or work, I seem to be _____, _____, and _____.

efficient	sluggish	precise
enthusiastic	competitive	determined
reflective	leisurely	thoughtful
placid	meticulous	cooperative

3. Socially, I am _____, _____, and _____.

outgoing	considerate	argumentative
affable	awkward	shy
tolerant	affected	talkative
gentle-tempered	soft-tempered	hot-tempered

4. I am rather _____, _____, and _____.

active	forgiving	sympathetic
warm	courageous	serious
domineering	suspicious	soft-hearted
introspective	cool	enterprising

5. Other people consider me rather _____, _____, and _____.

generous	optimistic	sensitive
adventurous	affectionate	kind
withdrawn	reckless	cautious
dominant	detached	dependent

6. Underline one word out of the three in each of the following lines which most closely describes the way you are

    a) assertive, released, tense   d) confident, tactful, kind

    b) hot-tempered, cool, warm   e) dependent, dominant, detached

    c) withdrawn, sociable, active   f) enterprising, affable, anxious

---

By permission of J. B. Cortes and F. M. Gatti, "Physique and Propensity," *Psychology Today* 4 (1970) 42–44.

TABLE 5–6.   Key to Self-Description Test.

ENDOMORPHIC	MESOMORPHIC	ECTOMORPHIC
dependent	dominant	detached
calm	cheerful	tense
relaxed	confident	anxious
complacent	energetic	reticent
contented	impetuous	self-conscious
sluggish	efficient	meticulous
placid	enthusiastic	reflective
leisurely	competitive	precise
cooperative	determined	thoughtful
affable	outgoing	considerate
tolerant	argumentative	shy
affected	talkative	awkward
warm	active	cool
forgiving	domineering	suspicious
sympathetic	courageous	introspective
soft-hearted	enterprising	serious
generous	adventurous	cautious
affectionate	reckless	tactful
kind	assertive	sensitive
sociable	optimistic	withdrawn
soft-tempered	hot-tempered	gentle-tempered

Key to Temperament Test: Count the number of adjectives that you selected in each of the three categories. For example if your totals are 10, 6, and 5, you have predominantly endomorphic traits; a 6, 10, 5 means you are high in mesomorphic traits.

By permission of J. B. Cortes and F. M. Gatti, "Physique and Propensity," *Psychology Today* 4 (1970) 42–44.

statement **13**

> **How you look to yourself and to others may differ and can affect your self-esteem.**

Introduction Each individual is different in body build and personality. However, the way a person feels about his body and how others perceive him or her is very important.

A recent study on the benefits of a jogging program in middle-aged men showed not only many beneficial physiological changes, but some improvement in various psychological parameters as well. Many of the psychological changes could be attributed to an improved image of self owing to an increased positive image of the body.[1]

This statement will attempt to increase the students' awareness of how their bodies look to others.

Procedure 1. The students will be videotaped performing the following suggested activities: three-sided pose, walking, walking a balance beam, weightlifting, and throwing and catching a ball.
2. The students should be assigned to small groups for the playback. After each member of the group has been viewed, a feedback session should be initiated utilizing the following questions:

   a. How would you rate yourself on the following scale in terms of your own body image? Mark the appropriate place on the scale with an **X**.

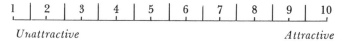

   Unattractive   *Attractive*

   b. How do you feel others would rate you in terms of their image of your appearance?

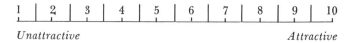

   Unattractive   *Attractive*

---

[1]A. H. Ismail and L. E. Trachtman, "Jogging the Imagination." *Psychology Today* 6 (1973), 78–88.

c. After viewing the tape, return to questions a and b and indicate where you rate yourself. Has your image of yourself changed?

d. After all members of the group have rated themselves, pass the scales around the groups and have each member rate the other members.

e. List the one part of your body which you found the most attractive.

f. List the part of your body which you found the most unattractive.

g. List several activities which you do regularly that you feel help to improve your self-image.

h. List several activities which you do regularly that you feel are probably deterimental to your body image.

Teaching Methods

Performance Objective

The student should be able to assess body image via the videotapes and respond to a series of questions.

Teaching Hint

Most videotaping takes about 1 minute per student, if the activities are well explained and organized sequentially. Groups of about five students (organized according to the series of taping) should be formed. Those five students should observe the tape, then meet for a feedback session following the suggested outline. The next group of five can view the tape, following the same format.

Materials

1. Videotape equipment.
2. Balance beam, balls, weights, etc. for activities.

statement **14**

How you look to yourself and others may be influenced by posture.

Introduction   According to Vitale,

> Good static and dynamic posture depends on good body mechanics in assuming various positions or performing certain actions. By good body mechanics, we mean the proper alignment of body segments and a balance of forces so as to provide maximum support, the least amount of strain, and the greatest mechanical efficiency.[1]

Most people generally do not become concerned with posture until poor body mechanics result in pain. Low back pain, a syndrome that affects about 30 million Americans, can be attributed to poor posture and weakened muscles that control the torso in about 80 percent of the cases, according to Dr. Hans Kraus.[2]

Although some medical evidence is available concerning poor posture and health, perhaps the major outcome of good posture is aesthetic. The students should not only examine posture statically as described in this statement, but should return to the body-image tapes and assess dynamic posture as well (Statement 13).

Procedure   Have the students, working in pairs, rate each other using the score sheet provided (Figure 5–7).

Teaching Methods   *Performance Objective*
    The student should be able to evaluate static posture utilizing the posture sheet.

Teaching Hints
1. Plumb lines can be constructed by attaching a nail, washer, or any heavy object to a string and hanging this overhead. The students

[1]Frank Vitale, *Individualized Fitness Program* (Englewood Cliffs, N.J.: Prentice-Hall, Inc., 1973).
[2]Hans Kraus and W. Raab, *Hypokinetic Disease* (Springfield, Ill.: Charles C. Thomas, 1961).

80

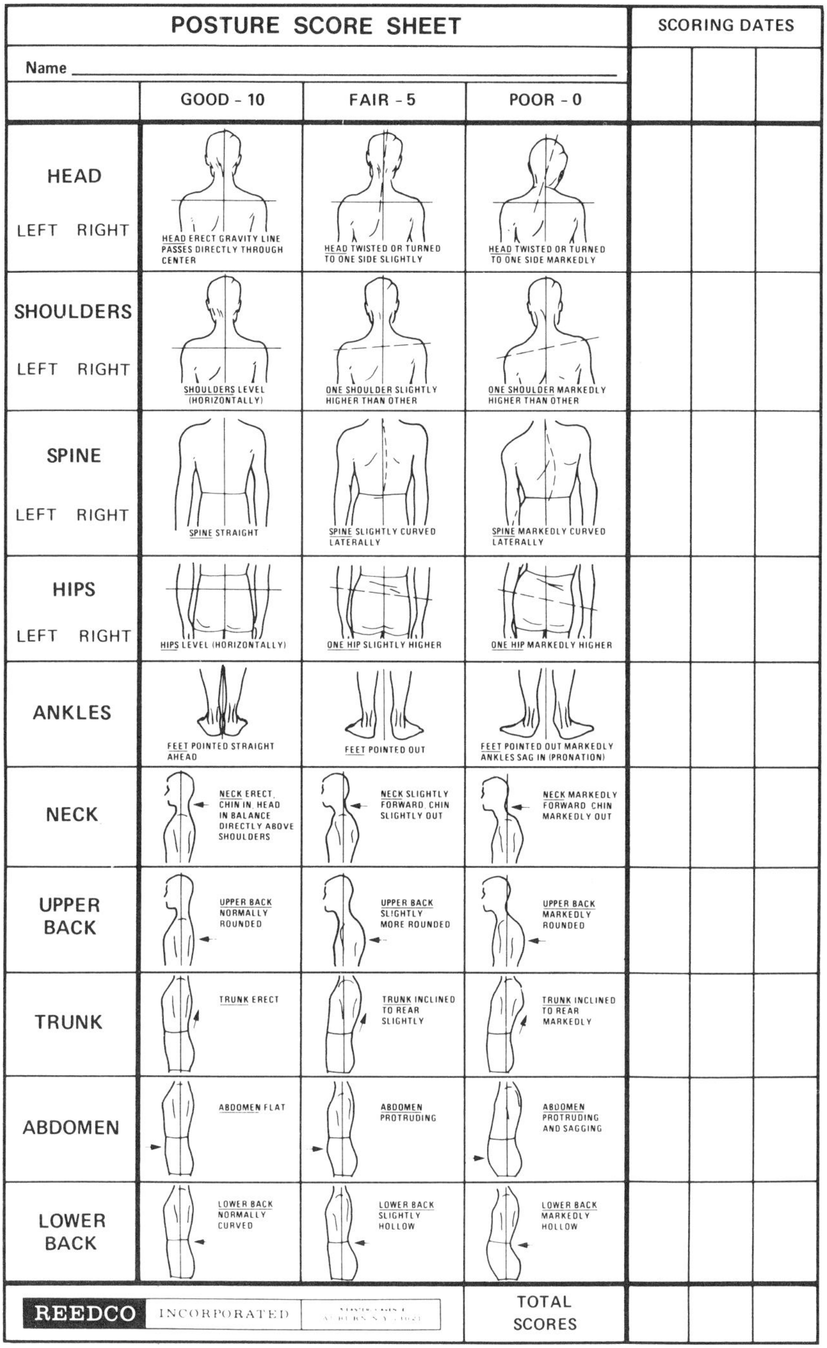

Figure 5–7. Posture score sheet. By permission of R. A. Hamilton and Reedco, Auburn, N.Y.

must carefully line up to the plumb lines while a partner uses the score sheet for evaluation.

2. An explanation of appropriate exercises for noted deviations and an analysis of proper posture can be obtained by reference to Vitale,[3] Van Huss,[4] or any other text discussing body mechanics, or by using the posture analysis form on p. 81. This is an excellent time to discuss proper body mechanics in general and the lower back in particular.

Discussion 1. List any deviations

Deviation   *Corrective Exercise*

a. _____   _____

b. _____   _____

c. _____   _____

2. Have the class discuss the question, "How important is good posture to you?"

Materials 1. Plumb lines.
2. Posture Analysis Form. (R. A. Hamilton, Reedco Incorporated Auburn, New York).

[3]Vitale, *Individualized Fitness Programs.*
[4]Wayne D. Van Huss et al., *Physical Activity in Modern Living* (Englewood Cliffs, N.J.: Prentice-Hall, Inc., 1969) .

chapter **6**

The Neuromuscular System

statement 15

> Movement may be limited by the degree of flexibility at a joint or series of joints.

Introduction Flexibility refers to the range of motion at a joint or series of joints. It can be a static or dynamic movement component relating to a particular joint, and involves both flexion and extension. Unfortunately, "general" flexibility tests do not exist. It is unacceptable to use one or two tests of flexibility and then state unequivocally that the results represent overall flexibility. Therefore when measuring flexibility we must choose a test or series of tests for the specific portion of the body.

In this statement the three flexibility tests the students will take are hip flexion, hip extension, and dynamic trunk rotation. These three tests were chosen because they are related to flexibility of the hip and back along with the elasticity of the hamstrings. It is possible that many cases of low back pain can be improved, if not cured, by a carefully prescribed program of stretching exercises to improve flexibility around this area. Lost flexibility is primarily the result of lack of movement and an excessive amount of time in a static position.

Procedure The students should take the following three tests and record their percentile scores from Tables 6–1 and 6–2.

   a. Trunk Flexion (see Figure 6–1a)
      1. Stand on a bench with the knees fully extended and the feet together.
      2. Bend forward, reaching toward the bench.
      3. Measure the point where the fingertips touch the measuring stick (do not allow bouncing motions).
      4. Record the distance.
   b. Trunk Extension (see Figure 6–1b)
      1. Lie prone on a mat with a partner holding the lower limbs.
      2. Rise from floor with the hands on the back of the neck.
      3. Hold for 3 seconds and measure from chin to floor.
      4. Record the distance.
   c. Dynamic flexibility (See Figure 6–1c)
      1. Stand two feet from a wall, facing away from the wall.

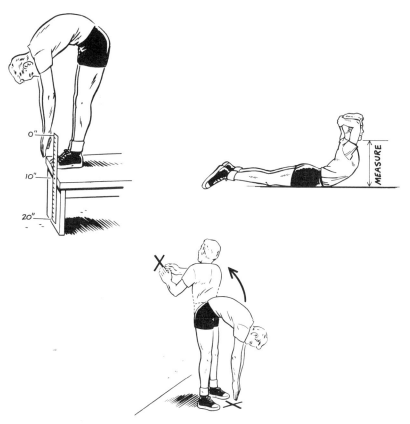

Figure 6–1. Flexibility tests. Adapted from Edwin A. Fleishman, *The Structure and Measurement of Physical Education*. (Englewood Cliffs, N.J.: Prentice-Hall, Inc., 1964).

2. There should be an X at the feet and an X on the wall about shoulder height.
3. Bend and touch the X between the feet and then rise and touch the X on the wall by twisting to the left: this completes one cycle. The alternate cycle is performed the identical way, twisting to the right.
4. Record the number of cycles completed within a timed 20-second period.

Teaching Methods

Performance Objective

The student should be able to determine the extent of trunk flexion, trunk extension, and dynamic flexibility by completing the given directions and performance standards.

TABLE 6–1. Dynamic Flexibility Norms.

Boys				Girls			
Age					*Age*		
14	*15*	*16–18*	*Percentile*	*15*	*16*	*17*	*18*
26	28	25	99th	25	23	20	20
25	26	24	98th	23	21	18	19
24	25	23	97th	21	19	17	17
23	24	22	95th	20	18	—	16
22	22	21	90th	18	17	16	15
21	21	20	85th	17	16	15	—
20	20	19	80th	16	15	—	14
—	19	—	75th	—	—	14	—
—	—	18	70th	15	14	—	13
19	18	17	60th	—	—	13	—
18	17	16	50th	14	13	—	12
17	16	15	40th	13	12	12	—
16	15	—	30th	—	—	—	11
—	14	14	25th	12	11	11	—
15	—	—	20th	—	—	—	10
14	13	13	15th	11	10	10	—
13	—	12	10th	10	—	—	9
11	12	11	5th	9	9	9	8
10	11	10	3rd	8	8	8	7
—	10	9	2nd	7	6	7	6
9	9	9	1st	5	3	6	—

Reprinted from Edward Fleishman, *The Structure and Measurement of Physical Fitness,* Englewood Cliffs, N.J.: Prentice-Hall, Inc., 1964, p. 112.

Discussion
1. List the possible flexibility tests that could be administered to assess total body flexibility.
2. List two physical activities and the joints involved in those activities.
3. What activity might be considered the best for promoting flexibility?
4. What occupations demand great flexibility?

Materials
1. Bench, Ruler
2. Dynamic Flexibility Norms
3. Norms for Extent of Flexibility of Trunk

TABLE 6–2. Test Norms for Extent of Flexibility of the Trunk.

Trunk Flexion	Trunk Extension	Percentile Rank
7.8	25.5	100
7.0	23.9	95
6.4	22.8	90
5.9	21.9	85
5.5	21.2	80
5.2	20.5	75
4.9	19.9	70
4.6	19.3	65
4.3	18.6	60
4.0	18.1	55
3.7	17.4	50
3.4	16.8	45
3.0	16.2	40
2.7	15.6	35
2.4	15.0	30
2.0	14.3	25
1.5	13.6	20
1.0	12.7	15
0.3	11.6	10
− 1.0	10.0	5
−3.5	7.0	0

From Richard A. Berger, *Conditioning for Men*. Boston: Allyn and Bacon Co., 1973, p. 93.

statement 16

> **The force of an isometric muscle contraction is related to the size of the muscle group.**

Introduction According to physiologists, a muscular contraction against a static resistance without a shortening or lengthening of the muscle is defined as an isometric or static contraction.

    The maximal force generated by a muscle during a static contraction is related to the cross-sectional area of the muscle, the number of muscle fibers that can be simultaneously contracted, and the mechanical advantage that comes from the joint angle and bone lengths.

    Most muscles consist of parallel fibers that contract along the long axis of the muscle. If we assume that a constant proportion of the fiber is contracted and if we measure at a constant joint angle, then the applied force will be directly related to the cross-sectional area of the muscle. This is true because the larger muscle has more or bigger muscle fibers.

Procedure
1. Measure the circumference of the upper arm.
2. Assess the isometric force by pulling against a fixed resistance as outlined in the Teaching Hints.
3. Individual results should be placed on a graph or chart.

Teaching Methods *Performance Objectives*
The student should be able to determine isometric force in the principal flexors of the upper arm and graphically identify the relationship between isometric force and an approximation of the circumference of the muscles involved

Teaching Hints
1. Suggested setup for the measurement of isometric force of the upper arm is shown in Figure 6–2.
2. For the above measurement a desk-type chair with the proper attachments or a table are appropriate. The student places the lower arm on the surface of the chosen piece of furniture and grasps the handle of the testing instrument. An angle of 90 degrees is recom-

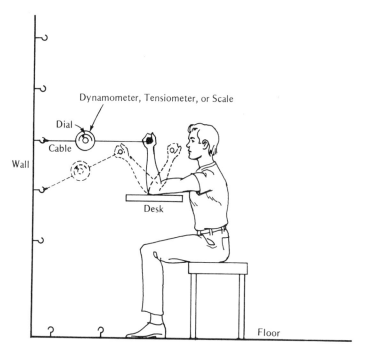

Figure 6–2. Determination of isometric strength at different joint angles.

mended to be established between the lower and upper arm. On the given signal a maximal force should be exerted by attempting a flexion movement around the elbow joint. Allow each student three trials and record the best of any one trial.

3. Measure the circumference of the upper arm at the mid-point between the elbow and shoulder joint with the muscle fully contracted.

4. The force exerted and the arm circumference for all students should then be placed on the following graph.

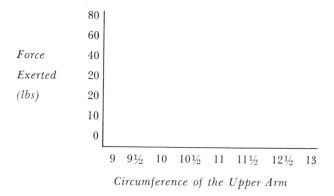

5. This statement and Statement 17 can be used together to compare the differences between muscle strength and muscle endurance.

6. Compare the ratio of the force exerted to the cross-sectional area. That is, calculate the force per square inch. To do this, remember that the area of a circle is equal to πr^2. (This is one technique to show that both the skinny and the muscular person may possess identical strength per unit of cross-sectional area of muscle.)

7. Sample calculation: If the measured circumference of the arm is 12 inches, the diameter of the arm can be estimated by using the following technique.

$$C = \pi d$$
$$12 = 3.14 \ (d) \qquad (12 \div 3.14)$$
$$d = 3.79 \text{ in}$$

If the diameter is 3.79, then the radius is 1.89 inches and the cross-sectional area is then calculated

$$A\,S = \pi r^2$$
$$A = 3.14 \ (1.89)^2$$
$$A = 11.21 \text{ sq in}$$

If the measured isometric force is 60 pounds, then the pounds exerted per square inch of cross-sectional area is 5.35.

$$\text{Force per sq. inch of cross sectional area} = \frac{\text{Force (lbs)}}{\text{Cross Sectional Area}}$$

$$= \frac{60 \text{ lbs}}{11.21 \text{ sq. in.}}$$

$$= 5.35 \text{ pounds per sq. inch.}$$

Discussion
1. Is strength related to the circumference of the upper arm?
2. How does your force per square inch relate to other members of the class?
3. How are muscle strength and muscle endurance related?
4. What are some of the possible sources of error in this experiment?

Materials
1. A table or desk-type chair.
2. A dynamometer, tensionmeter, or scales obtained from the industrial arts shop and a length of chain, wire, or rope with a handle.
3. A tape measure.

statement 17

Muscles have an endurance capacity to accomplish long-term tasks.

Introduction   Statement 16 discussed isometric or static contractions. This statement considers isotonic muscle contractions, which involve (1) a shortening of the muscle, (2) a range of motion, and (3) the performance of work. Endurance refers to the ability of the muscle to continue to perform work over an extended period of time.

    Statement 16 stated that the muscular force capable of being exerted is related to the size of the muscle involved in the contraction. Muscular endurance, on the other hand, demands an involvement of the circulatory system to deliver increased amounts of oxygen and glucose or fatty acids for energy production.

    This statement should allow the student to investigate the observable difference between muscular strength and muscular endurance.

Procedure   1. Measure the circumference of the upper arm with a cloth or metal tape measure, as was done in Statement 16.

2. Working in pairs, one student should stand with his back straight against the wall while holding a suitable weight, as determined by the instructor. The partner will stand at the side of the subject holding an object so that contact is made each time the subject performs a forearm flexion to a 90° angle. The subject should keep the rhythm determined by a metronome while raising and lowering the forearm. Each contact is considered one unit of work. When the subject does not perform the "lift" on two consecutive attempts, the exercise should be stopped; at this point the subject has probably reached the upper limits of work output or isotonic endurance.

Teaching Methods   *Performance Objective*

    The student should be able to determine a measure of isotonic endurance in the principle flexors of the forearm and plot the relationship between the circumference of the upper arm and work output.

91

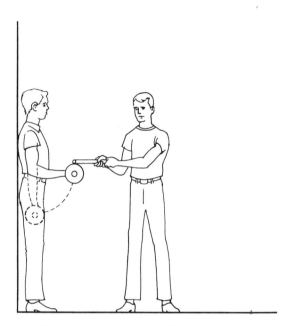

Figure 6–3. Measuring endurance capacity.

Teaching Hints
1. Use the same methods for measuring the upper arm as described in Statement 16.
2. The student should perform this task with the same hand that was used in Statement 16.
3. The method of performing the task is shown in Figure 6–3.
4. The instructor should select the weights in relation to the estimated endurance capacity of the class. (For high school students we recommend 15 pounds for males, 10 pounds for females; the work cycle should be about 60 repetitions per second.)

Discussion   1. Plot the following graph:

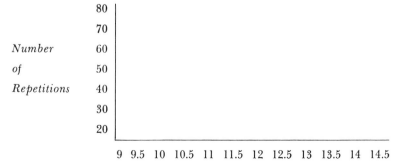

Circumference of Upper Arm (inches)

2. Is endurance related to the circumference of the upper arm?
3. Using the calculated information from the two graphs (in Statements 16 and 17), are strength and endurance the same?
4. Why did the subject stop lifting the weights?
5. What would happen if the weight were reduced? Increased?
6. Make a list of the factors involved in muscular strength and muscular endurance. How do these factors alter strength and edurance?

Factor	Muscular Strength	Muscular Endurance
1. _____	_____	_____
2. _____	_____	_____
3. _____	_____	_____
4. _____	_____	_____
5. _____	_____	_____

Materials   1. Metronome.
2. Weights.

statement 18

> **Muscle strength is related to the length of the muscle at the time of contraction.**

Introduction The amount of weight a muscle can lift depends upon the initial length of the muscle and the anatomical connections of the muscle to the bones. There are two reasons why you should be able to lift the least amount of weight when the arm is fully extended: (1) the angle of pull of the muscle is very poor, and (2) the muscle is at its longest physiological stretch length.

It is generally considered that for forearm flexion between 125° and 90° the angle of elbow flexion is at its optimal length for force generation. At less than 45° and greater than 160° the pull is not as efficient because the angle is poor and the muscle is close to its maximal physiological lengths for shortening and lengthening.

Procedure 1. The strength or force of the forearm flexors should be tested at the following angles on the dynamometer and recorded:

Angle	Force in lbs
160°	_____
125°	_____
90°	_____
45°	_____

2. The student should then complete the following graph:

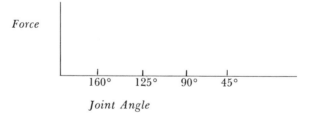

94

Teaching   *Performance Objective*
Methods   The student should be able to assess and plot on a graph the relationship between force exerted and the joint angle of the arm flexors.

Teaching Hints
1. This statement can be integrated with Statement 16 (the same
   equipment would be necessary). To determine the angle at the
   elbow joint, a movable protractor can be used.
2. See Figure 6–2 of Statement 16 for the correct testing procedure.
   At each angle of pull the cable must be adjusted so that the direction of the pull is along the axis of the cable.
3. Appoint a student to administer the test and an assistant to serve
   as a recorder. When each student has completed each of the four
   angles, this information should be plotted on the graph shown in
   the Procedure.
4. The tester must make sure the force is being applied by the biceps,
   and not by a pulling action initiated at the shoulder.

Discussion 1. What joint angle is the optimal in terms of force exerted?
                2. What angle would be optimal for other joints? Why?
                3. What would be your strategy for an arm-wrestling championship?

Materials   1. See Statement 16.
                2. A movable protractor or home-made angle-measuring device.

statement 19

> Muscle development programs can be designed to promote either muscular strength or muscular endurance performance.

Introduction For proper development of muscular strength or muscular endurance, the specific muscles must be properly "overloaded."* Berger suggests a starting weight between 80 and 90 percent of maximum for the greatest efficiency in strength development.[1] The trainee should gradually increase from five repetitions to ten repetitions per set. When ten repetitions have been reached, the load should be increased 5 percent and the repetitions once again returned to five. This procedure should be continued until the strength goals have been reached.

Training for muscular endurance involves an extended muscular activity period with a reduced weight resistance. We suggest using a weight equal to 50 percent of maximum strength. The number of repetitions should be twenty to sixty per set for three sets. Once the maximum number of repetitions have been reached, the weight should be increased.

Procedure 1. The student should determine the maximum amount of weight that can be lifted (absolute maximal strength) in any of several exercises (curls, military press, bench press, toe raises, bent-over rowing, squats, etc.).

2. Use the following formulas for determing starting weights:

$$\text{Starting Weight for Strength} = \text{Weight Lifted} \times 80\%$$

$$\text{Starting Weight for Endurance} = \text{Weight Lifted} \times 50\%$$

3. Have the student complete the following chart:

---

*By overload we mean that for a muscle to increase its strength or endurance it has to be working at or near maximal resistance or duration respectively. A muscle will only respond when stressed and furthermore the type of response is specific to the type of overload, i.e., increase the resistance for strength adaptations and increase the work duration or speed for endurance adaptations.

[1]Richard A. Berger, *Conditioning for Men* (Boston: Allyn and Bacon, Inc., 1973).

Exercise	Maximal Lift	80% Maximum	50% Maximum

Teaching Methods

Performance Objective

The student should be able to determine desirable starting weights for the promotion of both muscular strength and muscular endurance.

Teaching Hints

1. Have a series of weights available at 10-lb intervals ranging from 20 lbs to 120 lbs. With these weights available, the students can easily move through the procedures. Upon selecting an exercise (e.g., curls), each student will begin lifting weight which he thinks appropriate. If the weight is lifted, the student will move on to a heavier one until the maximum weight has been reached. If the student determines 80 lbs to be the maximal weight for the overhead press, using the formula in Procedure 2, 64 lbs will be the starting weight for the development of muscular strength, while 40 lbs will be the starting weight for the development of a muscular endurance training program. This information should be recorded on the chart depicted in Procedure 3.

2. Any of the commercially manufactured muscle development devices would make an ideal piece of equipment for the teaching of this statement.

Discussion

1. Have the students develop the chart described below:

Body Part to be Trained	Training Exercise	Starting Weight	Sets	Repetitions

2. Develop an eight-week weight training program. Identity the goal and justify the program through a discussion of the overload strategy.

Materials   Several sets of weights or a commercially manufactured device.

statement **20**

Development of health and fitness can be promoted by circuit training.

Introduction   Circuit training is a system of exercises designed to develop simultaneously all the health and fitness criteria as described in Statement 4 (Orientation to Exercise).

Unlike the development of muscular strength, circuit training sets a limit upon the time allowed to complete the routine of suggested activities.

The basic considerations for developing a circuit training program are:

1. The circuit should include activities which stress all major muscle groups.
2. The overload technique should be any combination of time, sets, and repetitions.

Procedure   1. The instructor should design a circuit with the aforementioned considerations in mind.
2. The student should participate through the circuit and complete the chart below. Time to complete: Set I . . . , Set II . . . , Set III.

Activity	Sets	Weight	Repetitions

Teaching Methods

Performance Objective

The student should be able to complete the circuit exercise as developed by the instructor and complete the charts which are suggested.

Teaching Hints

1. A suggested seven-exercise circuit which promotes the described health and fitness parameters:

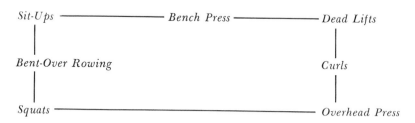

2. The circuit is designed to alternate muscle groups. The students should move through this set of activities as quickly as possible.

3. To determine whether or not the cardiovascular component is being sufficiently stimulated, the instructor should occasionally call for a pulse check. Take a 10-second count on the carotid artery and multiply by 6 to get the minute pulse count. If the heart rate is over 140 per minute, then a cardiovascular effect is considered to be occurring.

4. Another simple circuit that can be established utilizes free exercise and body weight. Several routines can be created to vary the activities. One procedure is to allow the students 5 seconds to change, with 20 seconds at each station. Directions can be given by the use of a tape recorder with appropriate background music during the exercise portion.

Routine A	*Routine B*
1. Bench stepping	1. Sit-ups
2. Sit-ups	2. Bench stepping
3. Chin-ups	3. Neck bridges
4. Toe touching	4. Rope jumping
5. Shuttle run	5. Push-ups
6. Job	6. Alternate toe touching
7. Squat thrusts	7. Jumping Jacks
8. Push-ups	8. Ladder walk
	9. Straddle and hurdle stretch
	10. Jogging

Discussion   1. Complete the following chart by listing the circuit exercises and checking which of the health and fitness criteria are being met by each exercise.

Health and Fitness Criteria	Exercises											Comments
Cardiovascular Capacity												
Flexibility												
Muscular Endurance												
Muscular Strength												
Body Composition												

2. Judging from the above information, does the circuit training method meet all of the parameters of health and fitness?

Materials   Weights or any commercially manufactured exercise machine.

statement 21

Low back pain is common and in most cases is avoidable.

Introduction Low back pain is a common problem in many people of all ages. But, according to Dr. Hans Kraus, 80 percent of all low back problems are a result of muscular weakness in the key muscle groups that support the torso.[1] Only about 20 percent of the low back cases are a result of the compression of the vertebrae.

The major muscle groups involved are in the back, abdominal, hip flexors, hip extensors, and the hamstring areas. This lower back syndrome is caused by a lack of strength and flexibility among the involved muscles and is often caused by a lack of physical activity, especially in occupations requiring long periods of sitting.[2]

The key to avoiding this "lower back syndrome" is to keep the trunk support and movement muscles strong and flexible.

Procedure 1. The instructor should lead the group through a variety of strength and flexibility exercises designed to prevent low back-pain problems (see Figure 6–4).

2. The students should complete the following chart:

Exercise	Muscle Group	Health and Fitness Criteria Stressed

[1]Hans Kraus and W. Raab, *Hypokinetic Disease* (Springfield, Ill.: Charles C Thomas, 1961) .

[2]Henry L. Feffer, "All About Backaches—Latest Advice from a Specialist," *U.S. News and World Report*, September 20, 1971, p. 74–78.

EIGHT EXERCISES RECOMMENDED BY DR. FEFFER

The following exercises are favored by Dr. Feffer to prevent back trouble. He recommends doing the entire set twice a day, performing each exercise four times in each exercise period at the start, increasing gradually to 10 times—but only after each individual has consulted his own physician.

LYING ON STOMACH

1. Pinch buttocks together. Pull stomach in. Hold position for five seconds, then relax for five seconds. Over a period of days, increase holding-relaxing period to 20 seconds.

LYING ON BACK

2. Bend knees with feet flat on floor, keeping arms at sides. Pinch buttocks together. Pull in stomach and flatten lower back against floor. Hold for five seconds, relax for five seconds. Gradually build up to 20 seconds.
3. Repeat exercise No. 2 with legs extended.
4. Draw knees toward chest. Clasp hands around knees. Keep shoulders flat against floor. Pull knees tightly against chest, then bring forehead to knees.

Exercise 4 (A)   *(B)*

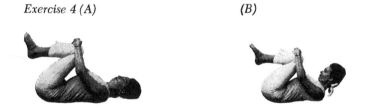

5. Bend knees with feet flat on floor; cross arms on chest. Raise head and shoulders from floor. Curl up to sitting position. Keep back round and pull with stomach muscles. Lower self slowly.
6. Bend knees, keeping feet flat on floor and arms straight forward. Touch head to knees. Lower self. Draw knees toward chest. Pull knees tightly against chest and bring forehead to knees.

Exercise 6 (A)   *(B)*

Figure 6–4. Exercises to prevent back trouble. By permission of Henry L. Feffer, "All About Backaches—Latest Advice from a Specialist," *U.S. News and World Report,* September 20, 1971, pp. 74–78.

(C) 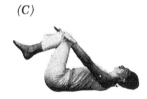   *(D)*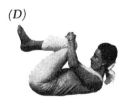

SITTING ON FLOOR

7. Keep legs straight. Pull stomach in. Reach forward with hands and try to touch toes with fingers. Use rocking motion.

SITTING IN A CHAIR

8. Place hands at edge of chair. Bend forward to bring head to knees, pulling stomach in as you curl forward. Keep weight well back on hips. Release stomach muscles slowly as you come up.

Teaching Methods

Performance Objective

The student should be able to perform the exercises for the lower back as described by the instructor and to complete the accompanying chart.

Teaching Hints

1. Mats should be placed on the floor for the students. The instructor should describe and demonstrate each activity.
2. The students should complete the exercises and state the muscle group involved and the health and fitness criteria promoted.
3. Students with bad backs should be excused from this exercise.

Discussion

1. What muscle groups seem to be involved in the exercises completed?
2. What health and fitness characteristics are promoted?
3. List two sports or recreational activities that might contribute to torso strength and flexibility.

Materials   Mats.

statement 22

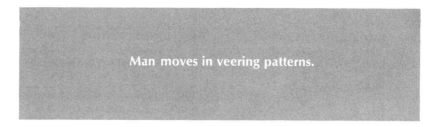

Man moves in veering patterns.

Introduction Schaeffer described a fundamental veering tendency in man, which he termed *spirokinesis*. He experimented by placing blindfolded subjects in a large field and having them walk, run, crawl, and drive automobiles. He also placed subjects in a large body of water and had them swim. The results of all these experiments were identical: man moves in circles. Schaeffer, however, was unable to explain this phenomenon.[1]

This statement will allow the students to create and test some theories about spirokinesis.

Procedure 1. The students should test this veering theory by experimenting with such activities as uprightness vs. crawling, carrying objects, gravitational pull, etc.
2. The students should take a practice walk on a designated line with and without blindfolds.

Teaching Methods *Performance Objective*

The student should be able to assess individual and class veering tendencies based on the experimental condition described.

Teaching Hints
1. Discuss the theory of veering, but let the students establish the theories to be tested.
2. A line 25 to 50 feet is long enough for the students to identify veering.

Discussion 1. Plot the results of the study on the following chart:

Start

[1]A. Schaeffer. "Spiral Movement in Man." *Journal Morphology*, 45 (1928), 293–398.

2. Does the veering pattern appear to the left-oriented, right-oriented, or "treelike"?

3. What physiological, anatomical, and psychological factors seem to be operating?

Materials   Blindfolds, a straight line in the gym or parking lot, and whatever materials the experimental condition calls for.

statement **23**

> **Skill in performance of an activity is dependent upon certain motor components.**

Introduction According to Johnson and Stolberg, motor performance parameters are defined as coordination, agility, power, balance, reaction time, and speed.[1]

The purpose of this exercise is to discover how these parameters become integrated in the learning of a new motor skill or in a sports performance. Are certain of these parameters more important than others, or are they specific to the skill being performed? Is it possible to assess these parameters? Can improvement be made with training in any of them? How do the health and fitness criteria differ from the motor performance parameters?

This statement attempts to discover more about these parameters, investigate the relationship between each of them, and to look at each parameter in terms of new skill learning.

Procedure 1. Administer as many as possible of the tests suggested below.

SUGGESTED TEST ITEMS:

Agility:
Shuttle run, as shown in Figure 6–5.

Power:
Standing broad jump, as described by the AAHPER Youth Fitness Test.[2]

Speed:
50-yard dash. See the AAHPER Youth Fitness Test

Reaction Time:
Use of a reaction timer would be the most accurate. For the purposes of this study, a ruler or yardstick dropped by a classmate

---

[1] Perry Johnson and Donald Stolberg, *Conditioning* (Englewood Cliffs, N.J.: Prentice-Hall, Inc., 1971).

[2] AAHPER Youth Fitness Test Manual, Revised ed. (Washington, D.C.: American Association for Health, Physical Education and Recreation, 1965.)

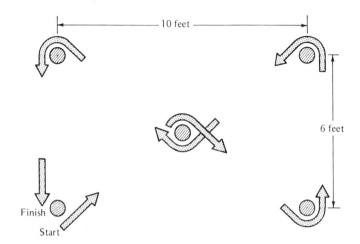

Figure 6–5. Shuttle run. Reprinted by permission of Perry B. Johnson, Wynn F. Updyke, Donald C. Stolberg and Maryellen Schaefer, *Physical Education: A Problem Solving Approach to Health and Fitness.* New York: Holt, Rinehart and Winston 1966, p. 427.

between the thumb and forefinger would suffice. (The reaction-time score should be given in inches in this case.)

Balance:

Several balance tests are available, such as walking on a 2 x 4 board forward, backward, and sidewards. Each time the subject places the foot on the floor it counts as an error.

Grip Strength

Although this is not a motor performance parameter by definition, it is interesting to relate one strength item to the others. A hand dynamometer is required. Any strength item could be used instead.

2. Record the results in the following table:

NAME	Shuttle Run	Balance	Grip Strength	Standing Broad Jump	50 yd Dash	Reaction Time

3. Assign individual students to discuss the relationship between any of these parameters of success in learning a motor skill.

Teaching Methods

Performance Objectives

The student should be able to compare individual motor performance parameters to established standards and to graph some relationships between the several parameters.

Teaching Hints

1. The instructor must decide which of these parameters are applicable in terms of facilities and equipment. The suggested tests are only for convenience. If the school does administer so-called "physical fitness" tests then these can be used. For example, the AAHPER Youth Fitness Test includes the parameters of speed, power, and agility with appropriate norms.
2. The administration of the tests can be accomplished with the aid of some selected class members or student leaders. Although these tests can be administered over a period of time, for best results in the understanding of this statement a single testing session is best.
3. The students should record the results of each test on a blackboard or master sheet. Selected students should be assigned to prepare a graph relating any two of the motor performance parameters. For example, balance related to speed could be examined by plotting the following graph:

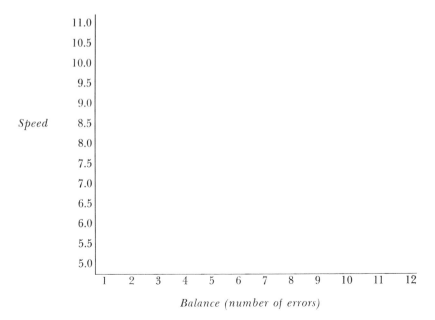

Balance (number of errors)

Discussion   1. What relationships were found between the various motor performance parameters? Are any of these parameters related to the learning of a new skill as outlined in Statement 24?
2. Discuss specificity and generality in terms of motor performance.
3. Are the items on your school's physical fitness test considered parameters of health and fitness or motor performance?

Materials   The materials will depend upon the local situation and the type of tests selected.

statement **24**

> **The process involved in learning a motor skill is dependent upon many factors.**

Introduction   The learning of a motor skill is sometimes a complicated and discouraging task. A simplified model of motor skill learning is offered in Figure 6–6, below.

This model indicates that some sensory input is initially involved: e.g., tactile, visual, auditory, kinesthetic, etc. In early skill learning, the sensory information is integrated in the brain. The activity in the brain makes possible an evaluation regarding the present stimulus and helps a person perceive the present information in terms of any past or current experiences.

In three-ball juggling the first stage is to toss the ball into the air. Although the brain recognizes that it has not stored any information on three-ball juggling, it does recognize the skill of tossing the ball into the air and catching it before the ball hits the ground. Once the brain has integrated the sensory information, the next step is to organize some type of output. The output in motor learning results in a muscular response. This response may be initially correct or incorrect. When the juggler tosses the ball into the air it may be a good throw that is just right or it may be a bad toss, thus classified as an incorrect response. To obtain a correct response requires that an adjustment factor be built into skill execution—this is labeled as "feedback." If this mechanism is working satsifactorily the next response will be closer to a correct one. Thus, the circuit continues until the skill is

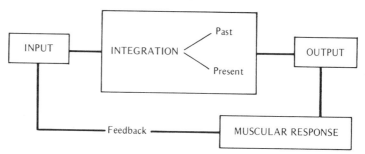

Figure 6–6.   Motor learning scheme.

111

fully imprinted in the brain and the resulting motor pathways (including the nerves and muscles).

Procedure
1. The instructor should introduce the class to a simple but entirely new skill, such as two- or three-ball juggling.
2. Each student should take a pretest. Holding the balls or beanbags, the student should attempt to juggle, counting the number of catches as the score.
3. The instructor should teach the skill, using demonstrations and practices.
4. After an appropriate number of practice sessions, each student should test himself. This score could consist of the greatest number of catches during any one of three trials.

Teaching Methods

Performance Objective

The student should learn a new skill and be able to list four factors necessary in new-skill acquisition.

Teaching Hints
1. If the instructor cannot juggle, another skill must be substituted. The skill may be an unusual skill or a commonly taught skill. The point is to get the students to think about possible models of motor learning. What physiological and anatomical systems are used? How do they relate to each other? The instructor should be more interested in the process of motor skill learning than in the actual skill acquisition.
2. Several uses can be made of this information for a better understanding of motor skill learning. For example, skill improvement can be related to the motor ability components identified in Statement 23. If plotted carefully, some understanding can be obtained regarding the general and specific nature of motor skills and motor ability components.
3. This lesson offers an opportunity for classroom research: for example, by assessing the whole vs. the part method of instruction, physical practice vs. mental practice, interference in early skill learning, sex differences, and skill performance vs. known scores on motor ability tests.

Discussion
1. How did you know how high to throw the ball?
2. What adjustments were made when the ball was transferred from one hand to the other?
3. What is the role of vision?

4. What did you think about when you started the learning process? Is the brain involved?
5. What role do touch and kinesthetic sense play?
6. List four sensory modalities involved in learning to juggle.
7. Can you draw a model of how one might learn a new skill?
8. List four factors involved in learning a new motor skill.

Materials   Balls or beanbags for juggling. If another skill is substituted those materials will be necessary.

chapter 7

Energy Systems

statement 25

The largest single expenditure of energy is the basal metabolic rate (BMR).

Introduction

The basal metabolic rate represents that amount of oxygen needed to sustain the lowest amount of cellular activity compatible with life. For example, if an individual should remain in bed for the day, the body would utilize the least amount of O_2 and produce the least amount of heat. This heat production is measured in units called calories. (Scientifically speaking, a kilocalorie is the amount of heat necessary to raise 1 kilogram of water one degree centigrade, specifically from 14°C to 15°C. This is the "calorie" referred to in future statements.)

Because the BMR accounts for the largest single daily caloric expenditure, it is important for a student to know his or her approximate BMR. Proper diet planning would be difficult without this information.

Procedure

1. Basal metabolic rate is determined by using the body surface area nomogram (Figure 7–1) and the heat production chart (Table 7–1).

TABLE 7–1.   Heat Production, Calories Per Hour Per Square Meter.

Age	Males	Females
6	52.7	50.7
8	51.2	48.1
10	49.5	45.8
12	47.8	43.4
14	46.2	41.0
16	44.7	38.5
18	42.9	37.3
20–24	41.0	36.9
25–29	40.3	36.6
30–40	39.5	36.6
40–50	38.0	35.3
50–60	36.9	34.4
60–70	35.8	33.6
70–80	34.5	32.6

Reprinted by permission of L.L. Langley, I.R. Telford and J.B. Christensen. *Dynamic Anatomy and Physiology*, New York: McGraw-Hill Book Co., 1969.

116

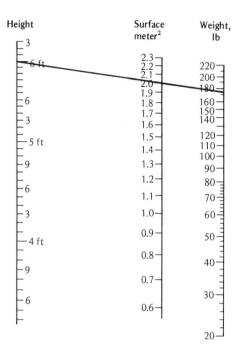

Figure 7–1. Body surface-area nomogram. By permission of L.L. Langley, I.R. Telford and J. B. Christensen. *Dynamic Anatomy and Physiology.* New York: McGraw-Hill Book Co., 1969, p. 661.

2. The student should first determine body surface area (BSA) by matching the height and weight columns in Figure 7–1 with a ruler; the intersection with the middle column gives the figure for BSA.
3. The second step involves the determination of heat production in calories per square meter. The student should locate this in Table 7–1 by finding the appropriate age and sex category.
4. The utilization of the following two-step formula is suggested:

Step 1. $\dfrac{}{\text{BSA}} \times \dfrac{}{\text{Heat Production}} = \dfrac{}{\text{Cal/hr/sq. meter}}$

Step 2. $\dfrac{}{\text{Cal/hr/sq. meter}} \times 24 \text{ hrs} = \dfrac{}{\text{BMR Cal/day}}$

Teaching Methods

Performance Objective
        The student should be able to determine basal metabolic rate using the tables and formula presented.

Teaching Hints

1. Carefully guide the students through the steps listed in the procedures. Most students have never used a nomogram, so its use must be explained carefully.
2. The BMR in cal/day should be immediately inserted into the appropriate space in Statement 26 beneath the *Expenditure* column.
3. Call for several students' BMRs and write them on the blackboard noting "male" and "female" beside the figure. Then call for observations about the list.

Discussion

1. What factors seem to determine basal metabolic rate?
2. Ask how many calories would a student spend if he remained in bed all day? How many calories of food would be necessary for that student to retain his present weight?

Materials   Table 7–1 and Figure 7–1.

statement **26**

> Gain or loss of weight is dependent upon balance of energy.

Introduction Energy balance is achieved when energy intake equals energy expenditure. To maintain a constant body weight, the daily or at least weekly energy balance must be maintained. A positive energy balance (intake greater than expenditure) for most people would result in a weight gain. A negative energy balance (intake less than expenditure) for most people would indicate a weight-loss condition.

 This statement should allow the student to determine energy balance for one day.

Procedure 1. The student should complete Table 7–2.

 2. The intake column can be completed from the information derived

TABLE 7–2. **Energy Balance Table**

	INTAKE		EXPENDITURE		
Meal	Calories		Activity	Cost/hr	Total Daily Calories
			BMR (from Statement 25)	_____	_____
Breakfast	_____		_____	_____	_____
Snack	_____		_____	_____	_____
Lunch	_____		_____	_____	_____
Snack	_____		_____	_____	_____
Supper	_____		_____	_____	_____
Snack	_____		_____	_____	_____
Total	_____				_____

in Statement 27. All food and drink should be totaled for the entire day.

3. The expenditure column can be completed by estimating activity above the BMR for one day. This information is presented in Table 7–3. The student should add to the BMR the estimated caloric cost of the physical activity. For all relative sedentary activities (e.g. sitting, standing, studying, driving, etc.) the student should use the

TABLE 7–3. Energy Cost of Selected Activities.

Activity	Cal/min/lb	Cal/hr/150 lb
Archery	.034	305
Badminton:		
Moderate	.039	350
Vigorous	.065	585
Basketball:		
Moderate	.047	420
Vigorous	.066	595
Baseball:		
Infield-outfield	.031	280
Pitching	.039	350
Bicycling:		
Slow (5 mph)	.025	225
Moderate (10 mph)	.05	450
Fast (13 mph)	.072	650
Bowling	.028	255
Calisthenics:		
General	.045	405
5BX	.098	880
Canoeing:		
2.5 mph	.023	210
4.0 mph	.047	420
Dancing:		
Slow	.029	260
Moderate	.045	405
Fast	.064	575
Fencing:		
Moderate	.033	300
Vigorous	.057	515
Fishing	.016	145
Football (tag)	.04	360
Gardening	.024	220
Gardening-Weeding	.039	260
Golf	.029	260
Gymnastics:		
Light	.022	200
Heavy	.056	505
Handball	.063	570
Hiking	.042	375
Hill Climbing	.06	540

TABLE 7–3.   Continued

Activity	Cal/min/lb	Cal/hr/150 lb
Hoeing, Raking,		
Planting	.031	280
Horseback Riding:		
Walk	.019	175
Trot	.046	415
Gallop	.067	600
Jogging:		
4.5 mph (13:30 mile)	.063	565
Judo, Karate	.087	785
Motor Boating	.016	145
Mountain Climbing	.086	775
Rowing:		
(Rec 2.5 mph)	.036	325
Vigorous	.118	1060
Running:		
6 mph (10 min/mile)	.079	710
10 mph (6 min/mile)	.1	900
12 mph (5 min/mile)	.13	1170
Sailing	.02	180
Skating:		
Moderate (Rec)	.036	325
Vigorous	.064	575
Skiing (Snow):		
Downhill	.059	530
Level (5 mph)	.078	700
Soccer	.063	570
Squash	.07	630
Stationary Run:		
70–80 cts/min	.078	705
Swimming (crawl):		
20 yds/min	.032	290
45 yds/min	.058	520
50 yds/min	.071	640
Table Tennis:		
Moderate	.026	235
Vigorous	.04	360
Tennis:		
Moderate	.046	415
Vigorous	.06	540
Volleyball:		
Moderate	.036	325
Vigorous	.065	585
Walking:		
2.0 mph	.022	200
3.0 mph	.03	270
4.0 mph	.039	350
5.0 mph	.064	575
Water Skiing	.053	480
Wrestling	.091	820

Adapted from Frank Vitale, *Individualized Fitness Programs.* Englewood Cliffs, N.J.: Prentice-Hall, Inc. 1973, p. 186–187.

estimated figure of .010 calories/min/lb of body weight. For example, a 150 lb. person studying for one hour would use 90 calories.

Teaching Methods

Performance Objective

The students should be able to determine a day's energy balance based on the difference between caloric intake and caloric expenditure.

Teaching Hints

1. Statements 26 and 27 should be undertaken together. The student can work in groups when completing Table 7–3. Allow class time for this undertaking.
2. An example of Discussion question c:
   A student has a negative energy balance of — 500 Cal/day. How many days will it take to lose 1 pound of fat (3500 calories)?

$$\text{Time to lose/gain 1 lb Fat} = \frac{3500 \text{ Cal}}{\text{Energy Balance}}$$

$$= \frac{3500}{-500}$$

$$= -7 \text{ (or 7 days to lose 1 lb fat)}$$

Discussion

1. Each student should answer the following questions:
   a. Do you have a positive or negative energy balance?
   b. What is your difference between intake and expenditure?
   c. If 3500 calories is equal to 1 lb of fat, how many days will it take for you to gain or lose 1 lb?
   d. Will you gain or lose weight on this diet?
   e. Subtract all the energy cost of physical activity from the expenditure column. How many calories is this? Do you now change from a negative to a positive energy balance?
   f. What is the role of exercise in the maintenance of desirable weight, regarding the energy cost of daily living?

Materials   Tables 7–2 and 7–3.

statement 27

Introduction Most people do not know whether or not their present diet is of proper nutritional quality. According to food scientists, the human diet each day must consist of carbohydrate, protein, fat, vitamins, minerals, and water if health is to be maintained.

The purpose of this statement is to determine if the diet is of proper quality based on the recommended daily allowances prepared by the U.S. Department of Agriculture.

Procedure 1. The student should record all food and beverage ingested for a typical day.
2. Using Table 7–4, prepared by the U.S. Department of Agriculture, record the amount of calories, foodstuffs (protein and fat), minerals, and vitamins and enter in Table 7–5.
3. The student should total each column in Table 7–5 and record the recommended daily allowances (RDA) line from the information provided in Table 7–6.
4. The final step is to determine the difference between the amount actually ingested and the recommended daily allowance. For each heading the student will place the numerical difference and indicate with (+) if above the RDA and (−) if below.

Teaching Methods *Performance Objective*

The student should be able to determine the quality of the diet in terms of calories, protein, fat, vitamins, and minerals for one typical day based on the U.S. Department of Agriculture standards.

Teaching Hints
1. This exercise will take some time. You can allow the students to complete the chart either in class or as a homework assignment. Remember that for one day, "If you eat or drink it, you chart it."
2. The Department of Agriculture tables must be made available to as

123

TABLE 7–4. Table of Food Values.

Values for prepared foods and food mixtures have been calculated from typical recipes. Values for cooked vegetables are without added fat. The following abbreviations are used: Gm. for gram; Mg. for milligram; I.U. for International Unit; Cal. for calories; Tr. for trace. Ounce refers to weight; fluid ounce to measure.

Food, and Approximate Measure	Food Energy Cal.	Protein Gm.	Fat Gm.	MINERALS		VITAMINS				
				Calcium Mg.	Iron Mg.	Vitamin A Value I.U.	Thiamine B₁ Mg.	Riboflavin B₂ Mg.	Niacin Value Mg.	Ascorbic Acid Mg.
A Apple, raw, 1 medium 2½″ in diam.	76	.4	.5	8	.4	120	.05	.04	.2	6
Apple betty, 1 cup..........	344	3.9	6.7	34	.2	370	.13	.09	1.1	3
Apple butter, 1 tbs.	33	.1	.1	3	.1	—	Tr.	Tr.	Tr.	Tr.
Apple juice, fresh or canned, 1 cup.......	124	.2	—	15	1.2	90	.05	.07	Tr.	2
Applesauce, canned unsweetened, 1 cup...	100	.5	.5	10	1.0	70	.05	.02	.1	3
sweetened 1 cup.............	184	.5	.3	10	1.0	80	.05	.03	.1	3
Apricots, raw, three........	54	1.1	.1	17	.5	2,990	.03	.05	.9	7
canned, sirup pack, 4 medium halves, 2 tbs. sirup...........	97	.7	.1	12	.4	1,650	.02	.03	.4	5
dried, uncooked, 1 cup (40 small halves)	393	7.8	.6	129	7.4	11,140	.02	.24	4.9	19
cooked, unsweetened, 1 cup (25 halves approx.)......	242	4.8	.3	80	4.6	6,990	.01	.14	2.8	9
cooked, sweetened, 1 cup (25 halves approx.)......	400	4.9	.3	78	4.6	6,860	.01	.13	2.9	10
frozen, 3 ounces...	70	.6	.1	9	.3	1,410	.02	.03	.4	3
Asparagus, cooked, 1 cup cut spears......	36	4.2	.4	33	1.8	1,820	.23	.30	2.1	40
canned, green, 1 cup cut spears......	38	4.2	.7	33	3.3	1,400	.11	.14	1.7	31
Avocado, raw, ½ peeled, 3½ × 3¼″ diam.	279	1.9	30.1	11	.7	330	.07	.15	1.3	18
B Bacon, crisp, 2 slices...	97	4.0	8.8	4	.5	—	.08	.05	.8	—
Bananas, raw, 1 large, 8 × 1½″...	119	1.6	.3	11	.8	570	.06	.06	1.0	13
Barley, pearled, light, dry, 1 cup...	708	16.6	2.0	32	4.1	—	.25	.17	6.3	—
Bean sprouts, Chinese, 1 cup...	21	2.6	.2	26	.7	10	.06	.08	.5	14

Adapted from "Composition of Foods—Raw, Processed, Prepared." U.S. Department of Agriculture, Handbook No. 8.

TABLE 7-4. Continued

Beans:										
Red kidney, canned or cooked, 1 cup	230	14.6	1.0	102	4.9	—	.12	.12	2.0	—
Other (including navy, pea bean—raw), 1 cup	642	40.7	3.0	310	13.1	—	1.28	.44	4.1	3
Baked—pork and molasses, 1 cup	325	15.1	7.8	146	5.5	90	.13	.09	1.2	7
pork and tomato sauce, 1 cup	295	15.1	5.5	107	4.7	220	.13	.09	1.2	7
Beans, lima immature, cooked, 1 cup	152	8.0	.6	46	2.7	460	.22	.14	1.8	24
canned, solids and liquid, 1 cup	176	9.5	.7	67	4.2	330	.09	.11	1.3	20
Beans, snap:										
green, cooked, 1 cup	27	1.8	.2	45	.9	830	.09	.12	.6	18
canned, drained solids, 1 cup	27	1.8	.2	45	2.1	620	.04	.07	.5	7
wax, canned, drained solids, 1 cup	27	1.8	.2	45	2.1	150	.04	.07	.5	7
Beans, soya (See Soybeans)										
Beef cuts, cooked:										
Chuck, 3 ounces without bone	265	22.0	19.0	9	2.6	—	.04	.17	3.5	—
Flank, 3 ounces without bone	270	21.0	20.0	9	2.6	—	.04	.17	3.5	—
Hamburger, 3 ounces	316	19.0	26.0	8	2.4	—	.07	.16	4.1	—
Porterhouse, 3 ounces without bone	293	20.0	23.0	9	2.6	—	.05	.15	4.0	—
Rib roast, 3 ounces without bone	266	20.0	20.0	9	2.6	—	.05	.15	3.6	—
Round, 3 ounces without bone	197	23.0	11.0	9	2.9	—	.06	.19	4.7	—
Rump, 3 ounces without bone	320	18.0	27.0	7	2.1	—	.04	.13	2.6	—
Sirloin, 3 ounces without bone	257	20.0	19.0	9	2.5	—	.06	.16	4.1	—
Beef, canned:										
Corned beef hash, 3 ounces	120	11.7	5.2	22	1.1	Tr.	.02	.11	2.4	—
Roast beef, 3 ounces	189	21.0	11.0	14	2.0	—	.02	.19	3.6	—
Strained (infant food), 1 ounce	30	4.9	1.0	3	1.2	—	Tr.	.06	.9	—
Beef, corned, canned:										
Lean, 3 ounces	159	22.5	7.0	18	3.8	—	.01	.21	3.0	—
Medium fat, 3 ounces	182	21.5	10.0	17	3.7	—	.01	.20	2.9	—
Fat, 3 ounces	221	20.0	15.0	16	3.4	—	.01	.19	2.7	—
Beef, dried or chipped, 1 cup	336	56.6	10.4	33	8.4	—	.12	.53	6.3	—
Beef, dried or chipped, 2 ounces	115	19.4	3.6	11	2.9	—	.04	.18	2.2	—
Beef and vegetable stew, 1 cup	252	12.9	19.3	31	2.6	2,520	.12	.15	3.4	15

TABLE 7–4. Continued

Food, and Approximate Measure	Food Energy Cal.	Protein Gm.	Fat Gm.	MINERALS Calcium Mg.	Iron Mg.	VITAMINS Vitamin A Value I.U.	Thiamine B₁ Mg.	Riboflavin B₂ Mg.	Niacin Value Mg.	Ascorbic Acid Mg.
Beer (average 4 pct. alcohol), 8 ounces....	114	1.4	—	10	—	—	Tr.	.06	.4	—
Beets, red, raw, 1 cup diced.............	56	2.1	.1	36	1.3	30	.03	.06	.6	13
cooked, 1 cup diced...................	68	1.6	.2	35	1.2	30	.03	.07	.5	11
Beet greens, cooked, 1 cup...............	39	2.9	.4	1*171	4.6	10,790	.07	.23	.6	22
Beverages, carbonated:										
Ginger ale, 1 cup......................	80	—	—	—	—	—	—	—	—	—
Other, including kola type, 1 cup......	107	—	—	—	—	—	—	—	—	—
Biscuits, baking powder, 1–2½" diam. ...	129	3.1	4.0	83	.2	—	.02	.03	.2	—
Blackberries, raw, 1 cup.................	82	1.7	1.4	46	1.3	280	.05	.06	.5	30
canned, sirup pack, 1 cup.............	216	1.8	.5	45	1.8	460	.03	.05	.5	16
Blanc mange (vanilla cornstarch pudding), 1 cup..............................	275	8.7	9.7	290	.2	390	.08	.40	.2	2
Blueberries, raw, 1 cup.................	85	.8	.8	22	1.1	400	.04	.03	.4	23
canned, sirup pack, 1 cup.............	245	1.0	1.0	27	1.2	100	.03	.03	.5	33
frozen without sugar, 3 ounces........	52	.5	.5	14	.7	200	.01	.01	.2	12
Bluefish, cooked, baked, 1 piece 3½ × 3 × ½"...........................	193	34.2	5.2	29	.9	—	.15	.14	2.8	—
fried, 1 piece 3½ × 3 × ½"...........	307	34.0	14.7	28	.9	—	.16	.16	3.1	—
Bouillon cubes, 1 cube.................	2	—	.1	—	—	—	—	.07	1.0	—
Brains, all kinds, raw, 3 ounces........	106	8.8	7.3	14	3.1	—	.20	.22	3.8	15
Bran (breakfast cereal almost wholly bran), 1 cup............................	145	7.2	2.0	56	6.2	—	.22	.23	11.5	—
Bran flakes, 1 cup....................	117	4.3	.8	24	2.0	—	.19	.09	3.5	—
Breads:										
Boston brown, unenriched, 1 slice 3 × ¾"	105	2.3	1.0	89	1.2	70	.04	.06	.7	—
Cracked-wheat, unenriched, 1 sl. ½" thick	60	2.0	.5	19	2.2	—	.03	.02	.3	—
French or Vienna, unenriched, 1 pound	1,225	36.8	12.3	109	3.2	—	.21	.28	4.2	—

1* Calcium may not be available because of presence of oxalic acid.

TABLE 7–4. Continued

Italian, unenriched, 1 pound	1,195	39.5	3.6	59	3.2	—	.23	.30	4.5	—
Raisin, unenriched, 1 slice ½″ thick	65	1.6	.7	18	.3	Tr.	.02	.02	.2	—
Rye, American, 1 slice ½″ thick	57	2.1	.3	17	.4	—	.04	.02	.4	—
White, unenriched, 4 per cent nonfat milk solids, 1 slice ½″ thick	63	2.0	.7	18	.1	—	.01	.02	.2	—
Toasted, 1 slice ½″ thick	63	2.0	.7	18	.1	—	.01	.02	.2	—
Whole wheat, 1 slice ½″ thick	55	2.1	.6	22	.5	—	.07	.03	.7	—
Bread crumbs, dry, grated, 1 cup	339	10.5	4.0	98	2.3	—	.24	.19	2.7	—
Broccoli, cooked, 1 cup	44	5.0	.3	195	2.0	5,100	.10	.22	1.2	111
Brussels sprouts, cooked, 1 cup	60	5.7	.6	44	1.7	520	.05	.16	.6	61
Buckwheat flour:										
Dark, 1 cup sifted	340	11.5	2.4	32	2.7	—	.56	.15	2.8	—
Light, 1 cup sifted	342	6.3	1.2	11	1.0	—	.08	.04	.4	Tr.
Buckwheat pancake, 1 cake 4″ diam	47	1.6	2.3	67	.3	30	.04	.04	.2	—
Butter, 1 tbs.	100	.1	11.3	3	—	1*460	Tr.	Tr.	Tr.	—
Buttermilk, 1 cup	86	8.5	.2	288	.2	10	.09	.43	.3	3
Buttermilk, 1 quart	348	34.2	1.0	1,152	.7	40	.35	1.74	1.1	13
C Cabbage, raw, 1 cup shredded finely	24	1.4	.2	46	.5	80	.06	.05	.3	50
cooked, short time, 1 cup	40	2.4	.3	78	.8	150	.08	.08	.5	53
Cabbage, celery or chinese:										
Raw, leaves and stem, 1 cup 1″ pieces	14	1.2	.3	43	.9	260	.03	.04	.4	31
Cooked, 1 cup	27	2.3	.6	82	1.7	490	.04	.06	.6	42
Cakes:										
Angel food, 2″ sector	108	3.4	.1	2	.1	—	Tr.	.05	.1	—
Foundation, plain, 1 sq. 3 × 2 × 1¾″	228	3.8	7.6	82	.3	2*100	.02	.05	.2	—
With fudge icing, 3″ sector	314	4.0	10.4	88	.4	2*100	.02	.07	.2	—
Fruit, dark, 1 piece 2 × 2 × ½″	106	1.6	4.1	29	.8	3*50	.04	.04	.3	—
Cupcake, 1 2¾″ in diam.	131	2.6	3.3	62	.2	50	.01	.03	.1	—
Iced layer cake, 3″ sector	241	3.9	4.6	88	.3	70	.02	.05	.2	—

1* Year-round average.
2* If fat used is butter or fortified margarine, the Vitamin A value would be 350 I.U. per square and 520 I.U. per 2-inch sector iced.
3* If fat used is butter or fortified margarine, the Vitamin A value would be 120 I.U.

TABLE 7-4. Continued

Food, and Approximate Measure	Food Energy Cal.	Protein Gm.	Fat Gm.	Calcium Mg.	Iron Mg.	Vitamin A Value I.U.	Thiamine B₁ Mg.	Riboflavin B₂ Mg.	Niacin Value Mg.	Ascorbic Acid Mg.
Cakes (continued):										
Iced cupcake, 1 2¾″ in diam.	161	2.6	3.1	58	.2	50	.01	.04	.1	—
Pound, 1 sl. 2¾ × 3 × ⅝″	130	2.1	7.0	16	.5	1*100	.04	.05	.3	—
Rich, 1 square 3 × 2 × 2″	294	3.8	13.3	79	.4	2*160	.02	.06	.2	—
Plain icing, 3″ sector	378	4.4	14.7	88	.5	170	.02	.07	.2	—
Sponge, 2″ sector	117	3.2	2.0	11	.6	210	.02	.06	.1	—
Candy:										
Butterscotch, 1 ounce	116	—	2.5	6	.5	—	.01	Tr.	Tr.	Tr.
Caramels, 1 ounce	118	.8	3.3	36	.7	50	.01	.04	Tr.	Tr.
Chocolate, sweetened milk, 1 ounce	143	2.0	9.5	61	.6	40	.03	.11	.2	—
Chocolate creams, 1 ounce	110	1.1	4.0	—	—	—	—	—	—	—
Fondant, 1 ounce	101	—	—	—	—	—	—	—	—	—
Fudge, plain, 1 ounce	116	.5	3.2	3*14	.1	60	Tr.	.02	Tr.	Tr.
Hard, 1 ounce	108	—	—	—	—	—	—	—	—	—
Marshmallows, 1 ounce	92	.9	—	—	—	—	—	—	—	—
Peanut brittle, 1 ounce	125	2.4	4.4	11	.6	10	.03	.01	1.4	—
Cantaloupe, ½ melon 5″ diam.	37	1.1	.4	31	.7	4*6,190	.09	.07	.9	59
Carrots, raw, 1, 5½ × 1″	21	.6	.2	20	.4	6,000	.03	.03	.3	3
Grated, 1 cup	45	1.3	.3	43	.9	13,200	.06	.06	.7	7
Cooked, 1 cup diced	44	.9	.7	38	.9	18,130	.07	.07	.7	6
Catsup, tomato, 1 tbs.	17	.3	.1	2	.1	320	.02	.01	.4	2
Cauliflower, raw, 1 cup flower buds	25	2.4	.2	22	1.1	90	.11	.10	.6	69
Cooked, 1 cup	30	2.9	.2	26	1.3	108	.07	.10	.6	34

1* If fat used is butter or fortified margarine, the Vitamin A value would be 300 I.U.

2* If fat used is butter or fortified margarine, the Vitamin A value would be 620 I.U. per square.

3* The calcium contributed by chocolate may not be usable because of presence of oxalic acid; in that case the value would be 11 mg. per ounce.

4* Vitamin A based on deeply colored varieties.

TABLE 7–4. Continued

Food										
Celery, raw, 1 stalk, 8″ long, 1″ wide......	7	.5	.1	20	.2	—	.02	.02	.2	3
Celery, raw, 1 cup diced..............	18	1.3	.2	50	.5	—	.05	.04	.4	7
Cooked, 1 cup diced..................	24	1.7	.3	65	.6	—	.05	.04	.4	6
Chard, cooked, 1 cup..................	47	4.6	.7	1*184	4.4	16,960	.07	.28	.5	30
Cheese:										
Camembert, 1 ounce..............	85	5.0	7.0	30	.1	290	.01	.21	.3	—
Cheddar, 1 ounce (1″ cube)........	113	7.1	9.1	206	.3	400	.01	.12	Tr.	—
Cottage from skim milk, 1 cup..........	215	43.9	1.1	216	.7	50	.04	.69	.2	—
Cottage from skim milk, 2 tbs	25	6.0	.1	27	.1	10	.01	.09	Tr.	—
Cream cheese, 1 ounce............	106	2.6	10.5	19	.1	410	Tr.	.06	Tr.	—
Limburger, 1 ounce.............	97	6.0	7.9	167	.2	360	.02	.14	Tr.	—
Parmesan, 1 ounce.............	112	10.2	7.4	329	.1	300	.01	.21	.1	—
Swiss, 1 ounce.............	105	7.8	7.9	262	.3	410	Tr.	.11	Tr.	—
Cherries, raw, sour, sweet, 1 cup pitted....	94	1.7	.8	28	.6	960	.08	.09	.6	13
Canned, 1 cup.........	122	2.0	.8	28	.8	1,840	.07	.04	.4	14
Chicken raw, broiler 2*, ½ bird (8 oz. bone out)	332	44.4	15.8	31	3.3	—	.18	.36	22.4	—
Roasters, 4 oz. bone out........	227	22.9	14.3	16	1.7	—	.09	.18	9.1	—
Hens, stewing, 4 oz. bone out......	342	20.4	28.3	16	1.7	—	.09	.18	9.1	—
Fryers, 1 breast, 8 oz. bone out......	210	47.0	1.0	28	2.2	—	.13	.18	21.1	—
1 leg, 5 oz. bone out.............	159	29.1	3.8	21	2.6	—	.14	.34	8.0	—
Canned, boned, 3 oz.............	169	25.3	6.8	12	1.5	—	.03	.14	5.4	—
Chile con carne, canned, ⅓ cup (without beans)............	170	8.8	12.6	32	1.2	130	.01	.10	1.9	—
Chili sauce, 1 tbs.	17	.5	.1	2	.1	320	.02	.01	.4	2
Chocolate, bitter, 1 ounce..........	142	1.6	15.0	1*28	1.2	20	.01	.06	.3	—
Sweetened, plain, 1 ounce......	133	.6	8.4	1*18	.8	10	.01	.04	.2	—
Chocolate beverage, 1 cup (made with milk)	239	8.2	12.5	260	.5	350	.08	.40	.3	2
Chocolate sirup, 1 tbs.	42	.2	.2	1*3	.3	—	—	—	—	—
Cider—See apple juice										

1* Calcium may not be available because of presence of oxalic acid.
2* Vitamin values based on muscle meat only.

TABLE 7–4. Continued

Food, and Approximate Measure	Food Energy Cal.	Protein Gm.	Fat Gm.	MINERALS		VITAMINS				
				Calcium Mg.	Iron Mg.	Vitamin A Value I.U.	Thiamine B₁ Mg.	Riboflavin B₂ Mg.	Niacin Value Mg.	Ascorbic Acid Mg.
Clams, raw, meat only, 4 ounces.........	92	14.5	1.6	109	7.9	120	.11	.20	1.8	—
Canned, solids and liquid, 3 ounces.....	44	6.7	.9	74	5.4	70	.04	.08	.9	—
Cocoa, breakfast, plain dry powder, 1 tbs.	21	.6	1.7	1*9	.8	Tr.	.01	.03	.2	3
Cocoa beverage made with all milk, 1 cup	236	9.5	11.5	298	1.0	400	.10	.46	.5	3
Cola beverage, carbonated, 1 cup........	107	—	—	—	—	—	—	—	—	—
Coconut, fresh, 1 piece, 2 × 2 × ½"......	161	1.5	15.6	9	.9	—	.04	Tr.	.1	1
Dried, shredded, 1 cup.............	344	2.2	24.2	27	2.2	—	Tr.	Tr.	Tr.	—
Milk only, 1 cup...................	60	.7	1.0	58	.2	—	Tr.	Tr.	.2	4
Cod, raw, 4 ounces edible portion.......	84	18.7	.5	11	.5	—	.07	.10	2.5	2
Dried, 1 ounce.....................	106	23.2	.8	14	1.0	—	.02	.13	3.1	—
Coffee, clear, 1 cup...................	—	—	—	—	—	—	—	—	—	—
Coleslaw, 1 cup.....................	102	1.6	7.3	47	.5	80	.06	.05	.3	50
Collards, cooked, 1 cup..............	76	7.4	1.1	473	3.0	14,500	.15	.46	3.3	84
Cookies, plain, 1 3" diam., ½" thick.....	109	1.5	3.2	6	.2	—	.01	.01	.1	—
Corn, 1 ear 5" long..................	84	2.7	.7	5	.6	2*390	.11	.10	1.4	8
Canned, solids and liquid, 1 cup......	170	5.1	1.3	10	1.3	2*520	.07	.13	2.4	14
Corn bread or muffins, 1, 2¾" diam.	106	3.2	2.3	67	.9	3* 60	.08	.11	.6	—
Corn flakes, 1 cup..................	96	2.0	.1	3	.3	—	.01	.02	.4	—
Corn flour, 1 cup sifted..............	406	8.6	2.9	7	2.0	4*370	.22	.06	1.6	—
Cornmeal (whole) cooked, white or yellow, 1 cup..............	119	2.6	.5	2	.5	5*100	.04	.02	.3	—
Corn sirup, 1 tbs.	57	—	—	9	.8	—	—	Tr.	Tr.	—
Crabs, canned or cooked, 3 oz. (meat only)	89	14.4	2.5	38	.8	—	.04	.05	2.1	—

1* Calcium may not be available because of presence of oxalic acid.
2* Vitamin A based on yellow corn; white corn contains only a trace.
3* Based on recipe using white corn meal, if yellow used, Vitamin A value is 120 I.U.
4* Vitamin A based on yellow corn flour, white corn contains only a trace.
5* Vitamin A based on yellow corn meal, white corn contains only a trace.

TABLE 7–4. Continued

Food										
Crackers, graham, 4 small	55	1.1	1.4	3	.3	—	.04	.02	.2	—
Saltines, 2, 2″ square	34	.7	.9	2	.1	—	Tr.	Tr.	.1	—
Soda, plain, 2, 2½″ square	47	1.1	1.1	2	.1	—	.01	.01	.1	—
Cranberries, raw, 1 cup	54	.5	.8	16	.7	50	.03	.02	.1	13
Canned or cooked sauce, 1 cup	549	.3	.3	22	.8	80	.06	.06	.3	5
Cream, light, table, 1 tbs.	30	.4	3.0	15	—	120	Tr.	.02	Tr.	Tr.
Heavy or whipping, 1 tbs.	49	.3	5.2	12	—	220	Tr.	.02	Tr.	Tr.
Cress, garden, cooked, 1 cup	73	7.6	2.5	380	5.2	5,940	.11	.23	1.3	52
Cress, water, raw, 1 pound (leaves & stems)	84	7.7	1.4	885	9.1	21,450	.37	.71	3.6	350
Cucumbers, raw, 1, 7½ × 2″	25	1.4	.2	20	.6	130	.07	.09	.4	17
Currants, red, raw, 1 cup	60	1.3	.2	40	1.0	—	.04	—	—	40
Custard, baked, 1 cup	283	13.1	13.4	283	1.2	840	.11	.49	.2	1
D Dandelion greens, 1 cup cooked	79	4.9	1.3	337	5.6	27,310	.23	.22	1.3	29
Dates, fresh and dried, 1 cup pitted	505	3.9	1.1	128	3.7	100	.16	.17	3.9	—
Doughnuts, cake type, 1	136	2.1	6.7	23	.2	40	.05	.04	.4	—
E Eggs, boiled, poached, 1	77	6.1	5.5	26	1.3	550	.05	.14	Tr.	—
Omelet, 1 egg	106	6.8	7.9	50	1.3	640	.05	.17	Tr.	—
Scrambled, 1 egg	106	6.8	7.9	50	1.3	640	.05	.17	Tr.	—
Yolk, raw, 1	61	2.8	5.4	25	1.2	550	.05	.06	Tr.	—
White, raw, 1	15	3.3	—	2	.1	—	—	.08	Tr.	—
Endive, Escarole, 1 pound raw	90	7.3	.9	359	7.7	13,600	.30	.53	1.8	49
F Farina, cooked, 1 cup	104	3.1	.2	7	.2	—	.01	.02	.2	—
Fats, cooking (vegetable), 1 tbs.	110	—	12.5	—	—	—	—	—	—	—
See also Lard, Oils										
Figs, raw, 3 small, 1½″ diam.	90	1.6	.5	62	.7	90	.06	.06	.6	2
Canned, sirup pack, 3, and 2 tbs. sirup	129	.9	.3	40	.5	60	.03	.04	.4	1
Dried, 1 large	57	.8	.3	39	.6	20	.03	.02	.4	—
Fig bars, 1 small	56	.7	.8	11	.2	—	Tr.	.01	.1	—
Flounder, summer and winter, 4 oz. (raw) edible portion	78	16.9	.6	69	.9	—	.07	.06	1.9	—
Frankfurters, 1	124	7.0	10.0	3	.6	—	.08	.09	1.3	—
Frog legs, raw, 4 oz. edible portion	82	18.6	.3	20	1.2	—	.16	.29	1.3	—

TABLE 7–4. Continued

Food, and Approximate Measure	Food Energy Cal.	Protein Gm.	Fat Gm.	MINERALS Calcium Mg.	Iron Mg.	VITAMINS Vitamin A Value I.U.	Thiamine B₁ Mg.	Riboflavin B₂ Mg.	Niacin Value Mg.	Ascorbic Acid Mg.
Fruit cocktail, canned, 1 cup (solids & liquid)	179	1.0	.5	23	1.0	410	.03	.03	.9	5
G Gelatin, dry, plain, 1 tbs.	34	8.6	—	—	—	—	—	—	—	—
Dessert powder, ½ cup (3 ounce pkg.)	324	8.0	—	—	—	—	—	—	—	—
Dessert, ready-to-serve, 1 cup	155	3.8	—	—	—	—	—	—	—	—
Ginger ale, dry, 1 cup	80	—	—	—	—	—	—	—	—	—
Gingerbread, 1 piece 2 × 2 × 2″	180	2.1	6.6	63	1.4	50	.02	.05	.6	—
Gooseberries, raw, 1 cup	59	1.2	.3	33	.8	440	—	—	—	49
Grapefruit, raw, ½ medium (4½″ diam.)	75	.9	.4	41	.4	20	.07	.04	.4	76
Grapefruit, raw, 1 cup sections	77	1.0	.4	43	.4	20	.07	.04	.4	78
Canned in sirup, 1 cup solids & liquid	181	1.5	.5	32	.7	20	.07	.05	.5	74
Juice, fresh, 1 cup	87	1.2	.2	20	.7	20	.09	.05	.5	99
Juice, canned sweetened, 1 cup	131	1.3	.3	20	.8	20	.08	.04	.5	87
Juice, canned unsweetened, 1 cup	92	1.2	.2	20	.7	20	.07	.04	.4	85
Juice, concentrate, frozen, 1 can, 6 fluid ounces	297	3.8	.8	63	2.4	60	.24	.13	1.4	272
Grapes, raw—Concord, 1 cup skins & seeds	84	1.7	1.7	20	.7	90	.07	.05	.3	5
Malaga, Muscat, 1 cup (40 grapes)	102	1.2	.6	26	.9	120	.09	.06	.4	6
Grape juice, bottled, 1 cup	170	1.0	—	25	.8	—	.09	.12	.6	Tr.
Griddle cakes (wheat), 1 cake, 4″ in diam.	59	1.8	2.5	43	.2	50	.02	.03	.1	Tr.
Guavas, common, raw, 1	49	.7	.4	21	.5	180	.05	.03	.8	212
H Haddock, cooked, 1 fillet 4 × 3 × ½″	158	19.0	5.5	18	.6	—	.04	.09	2.6	—
Halibut, broiled, 1 steak 4 × 3 × ½″	228	33.0	9.8	18	1.0	—	.08	.09	13.9	—
Ham, See Pork										
Hamburger, See Beef										
Heart, beef, lean, raw, 3 ounces	92	14.4	3.1	8	3.9	30	.50	.75	6.6	5
Chicken, raw, 3 ounces	134	17.4	6.0	20	1.4	30	.10	.77	4.4	5

TABLE 7-4. Continued

Food										
Herring, smoked, kippered, 3 ounces edible portion	180	18.9	11.0	56	1.2	—	Tr.	.24	2.5	—
Hominy grits, cooked, 1 cup	122	2.9	.2	2	.2	100	.04	.01	.4	—
Honey, 1 tbs.	62	.1	—	1	.2	—	Tr.	.01	Tr.	1
Honeydew melon, 1 wedge 2 × 7″	49	.8	—	26	.6	60	.07	.04	.3	34
I Ice cream, plain*, 1/7 of quart brick	167	3.2	10.1	100	.1	420	.03	.15	.1	1
J Jams, marmalades, 1 tbs.	55	.1	.1	2	.1	Tr.	Tr.	Tr.	Tr.	1
Jellies, 1 tbs.	50	—	—	2	.1	Tr.	Tr.	Tr.	Tr.	1
K Kale, cooked, 1 cup	45	4.3	.7	248	2.4	9,220	.08	.25	1.9	56
Kidney, beef, 3 ounces (raw)	120	12.8	6.9	8	6.7	980	.32	2.16	5.5	11
Pork, 3 ounces (raw)	97	13.9	3.9	9	6.8	110	.50	1.47	8.4	11
Lamb, 3 ounces (raw)	89	14.1	2.8	11	7.8	980	.44	2.06	6.3	11
Kohlrabi, raw, 1 cup diced	41	2.9	.1	63	.8	Tr.	.08	.07	.3	84
cooked, 1 cup	47	3.3	.2	71	.9	Tr.	.06	.06	.3	57
L Lamb:										
Rib chop cooked, 3 ounces without bone	356	20.0	30.0	9	2.6	—	.12	.22	4.8	—
Shoulder roast, 3 ounces without bone	293	18.0	24.0	8	2.2	—	.10	.19	3.9	—
Leg roast, 3 ounces without bone	230	20.0	16.0	9	2.6	—	.12	.21	4.4	—
Lard, 1 tbs.	126	—	14.0	—	—	—	—	—	—	—
Lemons, 1 medium	20	.6	.4	25	.4	—	.03	Tr.	.1	31
Juice, fresh, 1 tbs.	4	.1	—	2	—	—	.01	Tr.	Tr.	7
Lettuce, loose leaf, 1 head	32	2.6	.4	48	1.1	1,200	.10	.18	.4	17
Lettuce, loose leaf, 2 large leaves	7	.6	.1	11	.2	270	.02	.04	.1	4
Limes, 1 medium	19	.4	.1	21	.3	—	.02	Tr.	.1	14
Juice, fresh, 1 cup	58	1.0	—	34	.2	—	.11	.01	.3	65
Liver, beef, 2 ounces cooked	118	13.4	4.4	5	4.4	30,330	.15	2.25	8.4	18
Calf, 3 ounces raw	120	16.2	4.2	5	9.0	19,130	.18	2.65	13.7	30
Chicken, 3 ounces raw	120	18.8	3.4	14	6.3	27,370	.17	2.10	10.0	17
Lamb, 3 ounces raw	116	17.8	3.3	7	10.7	42,930	.34	2.79	14.3	28
Liver, canned, strained, 1 ounce (infant food)	30	4.5	1.1	7	2.0	5,440	.01	.61	1.8	—

* Based on 5 pounds of ice cream to the gallon, factory packed.

133

TABLE 7–4. Continued

Food, and Approximate Measure	Food Energy Cal.	Protein Gm.	Fat Gm.	MINERALS		VITAMINS				
				Calcium Mg.	Iron Mg.	Vitamin A Value I.U.	Thiamine B_1 Mg.	Riboflavin B_2 Mg.	Niacin Value Mg.	Ascorbic Acid Mg.
Lobster, canned, 3 ounces	78	15.6	1.1	55	.7	—	.03	.06	1.9	—
Loganberries, raw, 1 cup	90	1.4	.9	50	1.7	280	.04	.10	.4	34
M Macaroni, enriched, cooked, 1 cup (1" pieces)	209	7.1	.8	13	1.5	—	.24	.15	2.0	—
Macaroni & cheese baked, 1 cup	464	17.8	24.2	420	1.1	990	.07	.35	.9	Tr.
Mackerel, canned 1*, 3 ounces solids & liquids	153	17.9	8.5	221	1.9	20	.02	.28	7.4	—
Mangos, raw, 1 medium	87	.9	.3	12	.3	8,380	.08	.07	1.2	55
Margarine, 1 tbs.	101	.1	11.3	3	—	2*460	—	—	—	1
Marmalade, 1 tbs.	55	.1	.1	2	.1	Tr.	Tr.	Tr.	Tr.	1
Mayonnaise, 1 tbs.	92	.2	10.1	2	.1	30	Tr.	Tr.	—	—
Milk, cow: fluid, whole, 1 cup	166	8.5	9.5	288	.2	390	.09	.42	.3	3
Fluid, nonfat (skim), 1 cup	87	8.6	.2	303	.2	10	.09	.44	.3	3
Buttermilk, 1 cup	86	8.5	.2	288	.2	10	.09	.43	.3	3
Canned, Evaporated (unsweetened), 1 cup	346	17.6	19.9	612	.4	1,010	.12	.91	.5	3
Condensed (sweetened), 1 cup	981	24.8	25.7	835	.6	1,300	.16	1.19	.6	3
Dried, whole, 1 tbs.	39	2.1	2.1	76	—	110	.02	.12	.1	1
*Dried, nonfat solids (skim), 1 tbs.	28	2.7	.1	98	—	Tr.	.03	.15	.1	1
Malted beverage, 1 cup	281	12.4	11.9	364	.8	680	.18	.56	—	3
Half & Half (milk and cream), 1 cup	330	7.7	29.0	261	.1	1,190	.08	.38	.2	3
Chocolate flavored, 1 cup	185	8.0	5.5	272	.2	230	.08	.40	.2	2

1* The vitamin values are based on drained solids.

2* Based on the average Vitamin A content of fortified margarines. Most margarines manufactured for use in the U.S. have 15,000 I.U. of Vitamin A per pound; minimum Federal specifications for fortified margarine require 9,000 I.U. per pound.

* When a tablespoon or two of dry milk is added to a cup of skim milk, it makes the latter more pleasant to taste, and a good substitute for cream. Adds additional protein, vitamins and minerals too.

TABLE 7–4. Continued

Milk, goat, 1 cup	164	8.1	9.8	315	.2	390	.10	.26	.7	2
Molasses, cane, light, 1 tbs.	50	—	—	33	.9	—	.01	.01	Tr.	—
Medium, 1 tbs.	46	—	—	58	1.2	—	.06	.05	.4	—
Blackstrap, 1 tbs.	43	—	—	116	2.3	—	.01	.04	—	—
Barbados, 1 tbs.	54	—	—	—	—	—	—	—	—	—
Muffins, plain, 1, 2¾″ in diam.	134	3.8	4.0	99	.3	50	.02	.06	.2	
Mung bean sprouts, raw, 1 cup	21	2.6	.2	26	.7	10	.06	.08	.5	14
Mushrooms, canned, 1 cup solids & liquid	28	3.4	.5	17	2.0	—	.04	.60	4.8	—
Muskmelon, ½ melon 5″ diam.	37	1.1	.4	31	.7	6,190	.09	.07	.9	59
Mustard greens, cooked, 1 cup	31	3.2	.4	308	4.1	10,050	.08	.25	1.0	63
N Noodles, unenriched, containing egg, 1 cup (dry)	278	9.2	2.5	16	1.5	140	.15	.08	1.7	—
Cooked, 1 cup	107	3.5	1.0	6	.6	60	.05	.03	.6	—
Nuts:										
Almonds, shelled, 1 cup	848	26.4	76.8	361	6.2	—	.35	.95	6.5	Tr.
Brazil, shelled, 1 cup (32 kernels)	905	20.2	92.3	260	4.8	Tr.	1.21	—	—	—
Cashew, roasted, 1 ounce	164	5.2	13.7	13	1.4	—	.18	.05	.6	—
Peanuts, roasted, 1 cup medium halves	805	38.7	63.6	107	2.7	—	.42	.19	23.3	—
Peanuts, roasted, 1 tbs. chopped	50	2.4	4.0	7	.2	—	.03	.01	1.5	
Pecans, 1 cup halves	752	10.2	78.8	80	2.6	50	.77	.12	1.0	2
Pecans, 1 tbs. chopped	52	.7	5.5	6	.2	Tr.	.05	.01	.1	Tr.
Walnuts, 1 cup halves	654	15.0	64.4	83	2.1	30	.48	.13	1.2	3
Walnuts, 1 tbs. chopped	49	1.1	4.8	6	.2	Tr.	.04	.01	.1	Tr.
O Oatmeal or rolled oats, 1 cup dry	312	11.4	5.9	42	3.6	—	.48	.11	.8	—
Cooked, 1 cup	148	5.4	2.8	21	1.7	—	.22	.05	.4	—
Oils, salad or cooking, 1 tbs.	124	—	14.0	—	—	—	—	—	—	
Okra, cooked, 8 pods, 3 × ⅝″	28	1.5	.2	70	.6	630	.05	.05	.7	17
Oleomargarine, 1 tbs.	101	.1	11.3	3	—	460	—	—	—	—
Olives, green, 10 large	72	.8	7.4	48	.9	160	Tr.	Tr.	—	—
Ripe, Mission, 10 large	106	1.0	11.6	48	.9	40	Tr.	—	—	
Onions, mature, raw, 1, 2½″ diam.	49	1.5	.2	35	.6	60	.04	.04	.2	10

TABLE 7-4. Continued

Food, and Approximate Measure	Food Energy Cal.	Protein Gm.	Fat Gm.	MINERALS Calcium Mg.	Iron Mg.	Vitamin A Value I.U.	VITAMINS Thiamine B_1 Mg.	Riboflavin B_2 Mg.	Niacin Value Mg.	Ascorbic Acid Mg.
Onions, mature, raw, 1 tbs. chopped......	4	.1	—	3	—	Tr.	Tr.	Tr.	Tr.	1
Cooked, whole, 1 cup............	79	2.1	.4	67	1.0	110	.04	.06	.4	13
Onions, young green, 6 small............	23	.5	.1	68	.4	30	.02	.02	.1	12
Oranges, 1 medium, 3" diam.............	70	1.4	.3	51	.6	290	.12	.04	.4	77
Orange juice, fresh, 1 cup...........	108	2.0	.5	47	.5	460	.19	.06	.6	122
Canned, unsweetened, 1 cup...........	109	2.0	.5	25	.7	240	.17	.04	.6	103
Canned, sweetened, 1 cup............	135	1.5	.5	25	.8	250	.18	.05	.6	105
Orange juice concentrate, canned, 1 ounce	65	1.2	.2	17	.5	140	.10	.02	.3	63
Frozen, 1 can (6 fl. oz.)............	300	5.5	1.4	69	2.0	670	.48	.11	1.5	285
Oysters, meat only, raw, 1 cup (13–19 med.)	200	23.5	5.0	226	13.4	770	.35	.48	2.8	—
Stew, 1 cup (6–8 oysters)...........	244	16.6	13.2	262	7.0	820	.21	.46	1.6	—
P Pancakes (griddlecakes)										
Wheat, 1 cake, 4" diameter.......	59	1.8	2.5	43	.2	50	.02	.03	.1	Tr.
Buckwheat, 1 cake, 4" diameter........	47	1.6	2.3	67	.3	30	.04	.04	.2	Tr.
Papayas, raw, 1 cup, ½" cubes..........	71	1.1	.2	36	.5	3,190	.06	.07	.5	102
Parsley, common, raw, 1 tbs. chopped....	1	.1	—	*7	.2	290	Tr.	.01	.1	7
Parsnips, cooked, 1 cup..............	94	1.6	.8	88	1.1	—	.09	.16	.3	19
Peaches, raw, 1 medium.............	46	.5	.1	8	.6	880	.02	.05	.9	8
Peaches, canned, sirup pack, 2 medium halves, 2 tbs. sirup.......	79	.5	.1	6	.5	530	.01	.02	.8	5
Strained (infant food), 1 ounce........	17	.2	.1	2	.3	180	.01	.01	.2	1
Frozen, 4 ounces................	89	.5	.1	7	.5	590	.01	.03	.6	5
Dried, cooked, no sugar, 1 cup, 10–12 halves, 6 tbs. liquid.........	224	2.4	.5	38	5.9	2,750	.01	.16	4.3	11
With sugar added, 1 cup, 10–12 halves, 6 tbs. liquid...........	366	2.4	.6	37	5.8	2,750	.01	.15	4.3	12

* Calcium may not be available because of the presence of oxalic acid.

136

TABLE 7-4. Continued

Food										
Peanut butter, 1 tbs.	92	4.2	7.6	12	.3	—	.02	.02	2.6	—
Pears, raw, 1, 3 × 2½″ diam.	95	1.1	.6	20	.5	30	.03	.06	.2	6
Canned, sirup pack,										
2 medium halves, 2 tbs. sirup	79	.2	.1	9	.2	Tr.	.01	.02	.2	2
Strained (infant food), 1 ounce	15	.2	.1	3	.1	10	Tr.	.01	.1	Tr.
Peas, green, 1 cup	111	7.8	.6	35	3.0	1,150	.40	.22	3.7	24
Canned, 1 cup drained solids	145	7.2	1.0	51	3.4	1,070	.19	.10	1.6	15
Canned, 1 cup solids & liquid	168	8.5	1.0	62	4.5	1,350	.28	.15	2.6	21
Peppers, green, raw, 1 medium	16	.8	.1	7	.3	400	.02	.04	.2	77
Persimmons, raw,										
Seedless kind, 1, 2¼″ diameter	95	1.0	.5	7	.4	3,270	.06	.05	Tr.	13
Kind with seeds, 1, 2¼″ diameter	74	.8	.4	6	.3	2,570	.05	.04	Tr.	10
Pickles: Dill, 1 large	15	.9	.3	34	1.6	420	Tr.	.09	.1	8
Bread & butter pickles, 6 slices	29	.4	.1	13	.8	80	.01	.02	Tr.	4
Sour, 1 large	15	.7	.3	34	1.6	420	Tr.	.09	Tr.	8
Sweet, 1 average	22	.2	.1	3	.3	20	—	Tr.	Tr.	1
Pies: Apple, 4″ sector	331	2.8	12.8	9	.5	220	.04	.02	.3	1
Blueberry, 4″ sector	291	2.8	9.3	14	.7	160	.02	.04	.3	1
Cherry, 4″ sector	340	3.2	13.2	14	.5	530	.04	.02	.3	5
Custard, 4″ sector	266	6.8	11.3	162	1.6	290	.07	.21	.4	2
Lemon meringue, 4″ sector	302	4.3	12.1	24	.6	210	.04	.10	.2	1
Mince, 4″ sector	341	3.4	9.3	22	3.0	10	.09	.05	.5	1
Pumpkin, 4″ sector	263	5.5	12.5	70	1.0	2,480	.04	.15	.4	1
Pimientos, canned, 1 medium	10	.3	.2	3	.6	870	.01	.02	.1	36
Pineapple, raw, 1 cup diced	74	.6	.3	22	.4	180	.12	.04	.3	33
Canned, sirup pack, 1 cup crushed	204	1.0	.3	75	1.6	210	.20	.04	.4	23
Canned, sirup pack, 1 large slice &										
2 lbs. juice	95	.5	.1	35	.7	100	.09	.02	.2	11
Frozen, 4 ounces	97	.5	.2	16	.3	110	.07	.02	.2	22
Pineapple juice, canned, 1 cup	121	.7	.2	37	1.2	200	.13	.04	.4	22
Plums, raw, 1, 2″ in diam.	29	.4	.1	10	.3	200	.04	.02	.3	3
Canned, sirup pack, 1 cup (fruit & juice)	186	1.0	.2	20	2.7	200	.07	.06	.9	3
Popcorn, popped, 1 cup	54	1.8	.7	2	.4	—	.05	.02	.3	—

TABLE 7-4. Continued

Food, and Approximate Measure	Food Energy Cal.	Protein Gm.	Fat Gm.	MINERALS		VITAMINS				
				Calcium Mg.	Iron Mg.	Vitamin A Value I.U.	Thiamine B_1 Mg.	Riboflavin B_2 Mg.	Niacin Value Mg.	Ascorbic Acid Mg.
Pork, fresh:										
Ham cooked, 3 ounces without bone....	338	20.0	28.0	9	2.6	—	.45	.20	4.0	—
Loin or chops cooked, 1 chop........•	293	20.0	23.0	10	2.6	—	.72	.21	4.4	—
Pork, cured:										
Ham, smoked, cooked, 3 ounces without bone......•...	339	20.0	28.0	9	2.5	—	.46	.18	3.5	—
Luncheon meat: Boiled ham, 2 ounces....	172	12.9	12.9	5	1.5	—	.57	.15	2.9	—
Canned, spiced, 2 ounces....	164	8.4	13.8	5	1.2	—	.18	.12	1.6	—
Pork sausage, links, raw, 4 ounces.......	510	12.2	50.8	7	1.8	—	.49	.19	2.6	—
Pork, canned, strained, 1 ounce (infant food)	36	4.8	1.7	4	.5	—	.10	.08	1.3	—
Potatoes, baked, 1 medium, 2½" diam. ..	97	2.4	.1	13	.8	20	.11	.05	1.4	17
Boiled in jacket, 1 medium, 2½" diam.	118	2.8	.1	16	1.0	30	.14	.06	1.6	22
Peeled and boiled, 1 medium, 2½" diam.	105	2.5	.1	14	.9	20	.12	.04	1.3	17
French fried, 8 pieces 2 × ½ × ½" ...	157	2.2	7.6	12	.8	20	.07	.04	1.3	11
Hash-browned, 1 cup...........	470	6.4	22.8	35	2.3	60	.15	.11	3.3	14
Mashed, milk added, 1 cup...........	159	4.3	1.4	53	1.2	80	.16	.10	1.7	14
Mashed, milk and butter added, 1 cup..	240	4.1	11.7	53	1.2	500	.15	.10	1.6	13
Steamed or pressure cooked, 1 medium..	105	2.5	.1	14	.9	20	.12	.05	1.5	18
Canned, drained solids, 3–4 very small. ·;	118	2.8	.1	16	1.0	30	.11	.05	1.3	18
Potato chips, 10 medium, 2" diam. . ·	108	1.3	7.4	6	.4	10	.04	.02	.6	2
Pretzels, 5 small sticks...	18	.04	.2	1	—	—	Tr.	Tr.	Tr.	—
Prunes, dried, uncooked, 4 large........	94	.8	.2	19	1.4	660	.03	.06	.6	1
Cooked, no sugar added, 1 cup........	310	2.7	.7	62	4.5	2,210	.07	.20	2.0	2
Cooked, sugar added, 1 cup.........•■	483	2.9	.6	64	4.4	2,200	.09	.18	1.8	3
Prunes, canned, strained, 1 ounce (infant food)........	28	.3	.1	7	.4	210	.01	.01	.2	1
Prune juice, canned, 1 cup..........	170	1.0	—	60	4.3	—	.07	.19	1.0	2
Prune whip, 1 cup...........	200	3.8	.4	35	2.4	1,160	.05	.15	1.0	3

TABLE 7-4. Continued

Food										
Pudding, vanilla, 1 cup	275	8.7	9.7	290	.2	390	.08	.40	.2	2
Puffed rice, 1 cup	55	.8	.1	3	.3	—	.06	.01	.8	—
Puffed wheat, 1 cup	43	1.3	.2	6	.4	—	.01	.02	.6	—
Pumpkin, canned, 1 cup	76	2.3	.7	46	1.6	7,750	.04	.14	1.2	12
R Radishes, raw, 4 small	4	.2	—	7	.2	10	.01	Tr.	.1	10
Raisins, dried, 1 cup	429	3.7	.8	125	5.3	80	.24	.13	.8	Tr.
Raisins, dried, 1 tbs.	26	.2	—	8	.3	Tr.	.02	.01	Tr.	Tr.
Cooked, sugar added, 1 cup	572	3.2	.6	112	4.7	60	.18	.12	.6	Tr.
Raspberries, black, raw, 1 cup	100	2.0	2.1	54	1.2	—	.03	.09	.4	32
Red, raw, 1 cup	70	1.5	.5	49	1.1	160	.03	.08	.4	29
Frozen, 3 ounces	84	.7	.3	24	.5	70	.01	.03	.2	14
Rhubarb, raw, 1 cup diced	19	.6	.1	62[1*]	.6	40	.01	—	.1	11
Cooked, sugar added, 1 cup	383	1.1	.3	112[1*]	1.1	70	.02	.10	.2	17
Rice, brown, raw, 1 cup	784	15.6	3.5	81	4.2	—	.66	.05	9.6	—
Cooked, 1 cup	204	4.2	.6	14	.5	—	.10	.02	1.9	—
White, raw, 1 cup	692	14.5	.6	46	1.5	—	.13	.05	3.1	—
White, cooked, 1 cup	201	4.2	.2	13	.5	—	.02	.01	.7	—
White, precooked, dry, 1 cup	420	9.7	.2	4	.9	—	.02	.02	.1	—
Wild rice, parched, raw, 1 cup	593	23.0	1.1	31	—	—	.73	1.03	10.0	—
Rice, flakes, 1 cup	118	1.8	.2	6	.5	—	.02	.03	.3	—
Rolls, plain, pan rolls, unenriched (12 per pound), 1	118	3.4	2.1	21	.3	—	.02	.04	.4	—
Sweet, unenriched, 1	178	4.8	4.3	35	.3	—	.03	.07	.6	—
Rutabagas, cooked, 1 cup cubed or sliced	50	1.2	.2	85	.6	540	.08	.11	1.1	33
Rye flour, light, 1 cup sifted	285	7.5	.8	18	.9	—	.12	.06	.5	—
Rye wafers, 2	43	1.6	.2	6	.6	—	.04	.03	.2	—
S Salad dressings: Commercial, plain (mayonnaise type)[2*], 1 tbs.	58	.2	5.5	1	.1	20	Tr.	Tr.	—	—
French, 1 tbs.	59	.1	5.3	—	—	—	—	—	—	—

1* Calcium may not be available because of presence of oxalic acid.
2* Minerals and vitamins are calculated from a recipe.

TABLE 7–4. Continued

Food, and Approximate Measure	Food Energy Cal.	Protein Gm.	Fat Gm.	MINERALS Calcium Mg.	Iron Mg.	VITAMINS Vitamin A Value I.U.	Thiamine B₁ Mg.	Riboflavin B₂ Mg.	Niacin Value Mg.	Ascorbic Acid Mg.
Mayonnaise 1*, 1 tbs.	92	.2	10.1	2	.1	30	Tr.	Tr.	—	—
Salad oil, 1 tbs.	124	—	14.0	—	—	—	—	—	—	—
Salmon, broiled, baked, 1 steak 4 × 3 × ½"	204	33.6	6.7	—	1.4	—	.12	.33	9.8	—
Canned, solids and liquid:										
Chinook or King, 3 ounces	173	16.8	11.2	2*131	.8	200	.02	.12	6.2	—
Chum, 3 ounces	118	18.3	4.4	2*212	.6	50	.02	.13	6.0	—
Coho or silver, 3 ounces	140	17.9	7.1	2*197	.8	70	.02	.15	6.3	—
Pink or humpback, 3 ounces	122	17.4	5.3	2*159	.7	60	.03	.16	6.8	—
Sockeye or red, 3 ounces	147	17.2	8.2	2*220	1.0	200	.03	.14	6.2	—
Sardines: Atlantic type, canned in oil:										
Solids and liquid, 3 ounces	288	17.9	23.0	301	3.0	—	.01	.12	3.3	—
Drained solids, 3 ounces	182	21.9	9.4	328	2.3	190	.01	.15	4.1	—
Pilchards, Pacific type,										
Canned, solids and liquid										
Natural pack, 3 ounces	171	15.1	11.5	324	3.5	20	.01	.26	6.3	—
Tomato sauce, 3 ounces	184	15.1	12.6	324	3.5	20	.01	.23	4.5	—
Sauerkraut, canned, 1 cup drained solids	32	2.1	.4	54	.8	60	.05	.10	.2	24
Sausage: Bologna, 1 piece 1 × 1½" diam.	467	31.2	33.5	19	4.6	—	.37	.40	5.7	—
Frankfurter, cooked, 1	124	7.0	10.0	3	.6	—	.08	.09	1.3	—
Liver, liverwurst, 2 ounces	150	9.5	11.7	5	3.1	3,260	.10	.63	2.6	—
Pork, links or bulk, 4 ounces (raw)	510	12.2	50.8	7	1.8	—	.49	.19	2.6	—
Vienna sausage, canned, 4 ounces	244	17.9	18.6	10	2.7	—	.11	.14	3.5	—
Scallops, raw, 4 ounces edible muscle	89	16.8	.1	29	2.0	—	.05	.11	1.6	—
Shad, raw, 4 ounces edible portion	191	21.2	11.1	—	.6	—	.17	.27	9.6	—
Sherbet 1*, ½ cup	118	1.4	2.0	48	—	—	.02	.07	—	—

1* Minerals and vitamins are calculated from a recipe.
2* If bones are discarded, calcium content would be much lower. Bones equal about 2% of total contents of can.
3* Based on 6.8 pounds to the gallon, factory packed.

TABLE 7–4. Continued

Shortbread, 2 squares, 1¾ × 1¾″	81	1.1	3.9	2	.1	—	.01	Tr.	.1	—
Shredded wheat, 1 large biscuit, plain	102	2.9	.7	13	1.0	—	.06	.03	1.3	—
Shrimp, canned, 3 ounces drained solids	110	23.0	1.2	98	2.6	50	.01	.03	1.9	—
Sirup, table blends (chiefly corn sirup), 1 tbs.	57	—	—	9	.8	—	—	Tr.	Tr.	—
Soups, canned: 2*										
Bean, ready-to-serve, 1 cup	191	8.5	5.0	95	2.8	—	.10	.10	.8	—
Beef, ready-to-serve, 1 cup	100	6.0	3.5	15	.5	—	—	—	—	—
Bouillon, broth, and Consomme, ready-to-serve, 1 cup	9	2.0	—	2	1.0	—	—	.05	.6	—
Chicken, ready-to-serve, 1 cup	75	3.5	2.5	20	.5	—	.02	.12	1.5	—
Clam chowder, ready-to-serve, 1 cup	86	4.6	2.3	36	3.6	—	—	—	—	—
Cream soup—asparagus, celery, mushroom, 1 cup	201	7.0	11.7	217	.5	200	.05	.20	.1	—
Noodle, rice or barley, 1 cup	117	6.0	4.5	82	.2	30	.02	.05	.7	—
Pea, ready-to-serve, 1 cup	141	6.4	2.0	32	1.5	440	.17	.07	1.2	5
Tomato, ready-to-serve, 1 cup	90	2.2	2.2	24	1.0	1,230	.02	.10	.7	10
Vegetable, ready-to-serve, 1 cup	82	4.2	1.8	32	.8	—	.05	.08	1.0	8
Vegetable, strained, 1 ounce (infant food)	12	.7	.1	7	.3	700	.02	.02	.1	Tr.
Soybeans, whole, mature, dried, 1 cup	695	73.3	38.0	477	16.8	230	2.25	.65	4.9	Tr.
Soybean flour, medium fat, 1 cup stirred	232	37.4	5.7	215	11.4	100	.72	.30	2.3	—
Soybean sprouts, raw, 1 cup	49	6.6	1.5	51	1.1	190	.24	.21	.9	14
Spaghetti, dry, unenriched, 1 cup 2″ pieces	354	12.0	1.3	21	1.4	—	.09	.06	1.9	—
Cooked, 1 cup	218	7.4	.9	13	.9	—	.03	.02	.7	—
Spinach, raw, 4 ounces edible portion	22	2.6	.3	2*92	3.4	10,680	.13	.23	.7	67
Cooked, 1 cup	46	5.6	1.1	2*223	3.6	21,200	.14	.36	1.1	54
Strained (infant food), 1 ounce	4	.5	.1	2*22	.4	1,190	.01	.03	.1	2
Squash, summer, cooked, 1 cup diced	34	1.3	.2	32	.8	550	.08	.15	1.3	23
Winter, baked, mashed, 1 cup	97	3.9	.8	49	1.6	12,690	.10	.31	1.2	14
Winter, canned, strained, 1 ounce (infant food)	8	.3	.1	9	.1	560	.01	.02	.1	1

1* All ready-to-serve soups are calculated from equal weights of the condensed soup and water except cream soup which was based on equal weights of the condensed soup and milk.

2* Calcium may not be available because of presence of oxalic acid.

141

TABLE 7-4. Continued

Food, and Approximate Measure	Food Energy Cal.	Protein Gm.	Fat Gm.	MINERALS Calcium Mg.	Iron Mg.	VITAMINS Vitamin A Value I.U.	Thiamine B_1 Mg.	Riboflavin B_2 Mg.	Niacin Value Mg.	Ascorbic Acid Mg.
Starch, pure (corn), 1 tbs.	29	—	—	—	—	—	—	—	—	—
Strawberries, raw, 1 cup capped.........	54	1.2	.7	42	1.2	90	.04	.10	.4	89
Frozen, 3 ounces......................	90	.5	.3	19	.5	30	.02	.04	.2	35
Sugars:										
Granulated, cane or beet, 1 cup........	770	—	—	—	—	—	—	—	—	—
1 teaspoon........................	16	—	—	—	—	—	—	—	—	—
1 lump 1⅛ × ⅝ × ⅛″...............	27	—	—	—	—	—	—	—	—	—
Powdered, 1 cup (stirred before measuring).........................	493	—	—	—	—	—	—	—	—	—
1 tbs.	31	—	—	—	—	—	—	—	—	—
Brown, 1 cup (firm-packed).............	813	—	—	2*167	5.7	—	—	—	—	—
1 tbs.	51	—	—	2* 10	.4	—	—	—	—	—
Maple, 1 piece 1¾ × 1¼ × ½″.........	104	—	—	—	—	—	—	—	—	—
Sweet potatoes, baked, 1, 5 × 2″.......	183	2.6	1.1	44	1.1	3*11,410	.12	.08	.9	28
Boiled, 1, 5 × 2½″..................	252	3.7	1.4	62	1.4	3*15,780	.18	.11	1.3	41
Candied, 1 small.....................	314	2.6	6.3	63	1.6	3*10,940	.07	.07	.9	16
Canned, 1 cup.......................	233	4.4	.2	54	1.7	19,300	.12	.09	1.1	31
Swordfish, broiled, 1 steak 3 × 3 × ½″..	223	34.2	8.5	25	1.4	2,880	.06	.07	12.9	—
T Tangerine, 1 medium...............	35	.6	.2	27	.3	340	.06	.02	.2	25
Juice, unsweetened, 1 cup............	95	2.2	.7	47	.5	1,040	.17	.06	.6	75
Tapioca, dry granulated quick cooking, stirred, 1 cup......................	547	.9	.3	18	1.5	—	—	—	—	—
Tomatoes, raw, 1 medium, 2 × 2½″	30	1.5	.4	16	.9	1,640	.08	.06	.8	35
Canned or cooked, 1 cup.............	46	2.4	.5	27	1.5	2,540	.14	.08	1.7	40
Juice, canned, 1 cup.................	50	2.4	.5	17	1.0	2,540	.12	.07	1.8	38
Tomato catsup, 1 tbs.	17	.3	.1	2	.1	320	.02	.01	.4	2

2* Calcium based on dark brown sugar; value would be lower for light brown sugar.
3* If very pale varieties only were used, the Vitamin A value would be very much lower.

TABLE 7-4. Continued

Food										
Tomato puree, canned, 1 cup	90	4.5	1.2	27	2.7	4,680	.22	.17	4.5	69
Tongue, beef, medium fat, raw, 4 ounces	235	18.6	17.0	10	3.2	—	.14	.33	5.7	—
Tortillas, 1, 5″ diameter	50	1.2	.6	22	.4	1* 40	.04	.01	.2	—
Tuna fish, canned, 3 oz. solids & liquid	247	20.2	17.8	6	1.0	180	.04	.08	9.1	—
Tuna fish, canned, 3 oz. drained solids	169	24.7	7.0	7	1.2	70	.04	.10	10.9	—
Turkey, medium fat, raw, 4 oz. edible portion	304	22.8	22.9	26	4.3	Tr.	.10	.16	9.1	—
Turnips, raw, 1 cup diced	43	1.5	.3	54	.7	Tr.	.07	.09	.6	38
Cooked, 1 cup diced	42	1.2	.3	62	.8	Tr.	.06	.09	.6	28
Turnip greens, cooked, 1 cup	43	4.2	.6	376	3.5	15,370	.09	.59	1.0	87
V Veal, cooked, cutlet, 3 ounces without bone	184	24.0	9.0	10	3.0	2* —	2* .07	2* .24	2* 5.2	—
Shoulder roast, 3 ounces without bone	193	24.0	10.0	10	3.1	—	.11	.27	6.7	—
Stew meat, 3 ounces without bone	252	21.0	18.0	9	2.6	—	.04	.20	3.9	—
Veal, canned, strained, 1 ounce (infant food)	24	4.5	.5	4	.5	—	.01	.09	1.6	—
Vinegar, 1 tbs.	2	—	—	1	.1	—	—	—	—	—
W Waffles, 1	216	7.0	8.0	144	.8	270	.05	.14	.3	—
Watercress, raw, 1 pound (leaves & stems)	84	7.7	1.4	885	9.1	21,450	.37	.71	3.6	350
Watermelon, ½ slice ¾ × 10″	45	.8	.3	11	.3	950	.08	.08	.3	10
Wheat flour, whole, 1 cup stirred	400	16.0	2.4	49	4.0	—	.66	.14	5.2	—
Wheat products: Breakfast flakes, 1 cup	125	3.8	.6	16	1.0	—	.03	.06	1.7	—
Puffed, 1 cup	43	1.0	.2	6	.4	—	.01	.02	.6	—
Rolled, cooked, 1 cup	177	5.0	.9	19	1.7	—	.17	.06	2.1	—
Shredded, plain, 1 small biscuit 2½ × 2″	79	2.0	.6	10	.8	—	.05	.03	1.0	—
Whole meal, cooked, 1 cup	175	6.6	.7	22	1.7	—	.25	.08	2.3	—
Wheat germ, 1 cup stirred	246	17.1	6.8	57	5.5	—	1.39	.54	3.1	—
White sauce, medium, 1 cup	429	10.0	33.1	305	.3	1,350	.09	.41	.3	1
Wild rice, parched, raw, 1 cup	593	23.0	1.1	31	—	—	.73	1.03	10.0	—
Y Yeast, dried, brewer's, 1 tbs.	22	3.0	.1	8	1.5	—	.78	.44	2.9	—
Yogurt, commercial made with whole milk, 1 cup	170	11.0	8.0	560	.2	380	.10	.45	—	3

1* Vitamin A value of tortillas made from yellow corn; tortillas made from white corn have no Vitamin A value.
2* Data assumes cut to be prepared by braising or pot roasting.

TABLE 7–5. Diet Composition Calculation Table

Meal	Diet Constituents										
	Calories	Protein	Fat	CHO	Calcium	Iron	Vit A	Vit B$_1$	Vit B$_2$	Niacin	Vit C
Breakfast											
Lunch											
Dinner											
Snacks											
Total											
RDA											

many students as possible. Students can work in groups. Many of the ingested foods and the quantity will be similar.

3. This statement integrates well with Statements 26 and 29.

Discussion

1. Does your diet always contain the same number of calories, foodstuffs, vitamins, and minerals found for the day that was charted? If not, what was different for this particular day? How long would a deficiency in a particular vitamin take to impair health?

2. Compare your total for the day to the RDA.

3. Did you discover a deficiency in any one of the foodstuffs, vitamins, or minerals?

4. What types of and amount of foods are needed to return this deficiency to above the RDA?

5. What changes are necessary to improve the quality of your diet?

Materials Tables 7–4, 7–5, and 7–6.

TABLE 7–6. Recommended Dietary Allowances, from National Research Council, 1968.

The allowance levels are intended to cover individual variations among most normal persons as they live in the United States under usual environmental stresses. The recommended allowances can be attained with a variety of common foods, providing other nutrients for which human requirements have been less well defined.
The following abbreviations are used: Gm. for gram; Mg. for milligram; I.U. for International Unit

Family Members	Weight Pounds	Height Feet Inches	Calories	Protein Gms.	Calcium Gms.	Iron Mg.	Vitamin A I.U.	Thiamine Mg.	Riboflavin Mg.	Niacin* Mg. Equiv.	Asc. Acid Mg.	Vitamin D I.U.
Men:												
18–35 years	154	5–9	2,900	70	0.8	10	5,000	1.2	1.7	19	70	
35–55 years	154	5–9	2,600	70	0.8	10	5,000	1.0	1.6	17	70	
55–75 years	154	5–9	2,200	70	0.8	10	5,000	0.9	1.3	15	70	
Women:												
18–35 years	128	5–4	2,100	58	0.8	15	5,000	0.8	1.3	14	70	
35–55 years	128	5–4	1,900	58	0.8	15	5,000	0.8	1.2	13	70	
55–75 years	128	5–4	1,600	58	0.8	10	5,000	0.8	1.2	13	70	
Pregnant (2nd and 3rd trimester)			+ 200	+20	+0.5	+5	+1,000	+0.2	+0.3	+3	+30	400
Lactating			+1,000	+40	+0.5	+5	+3,000	+0.4	+0.6	+7	+30	400
Children:												
1–3 years	29	2–10	1,300	32	0.8	8	2,000	0.5	0.8	9	40	400
3–6 years	40	3–6	1,600	40	0.8	10	2,500	0.6	1.0	11	50	400
6–9 years	53	4–1	2,100	52	0.8	12	3,500	0.8	1.3	14	60	400
Boys:												
9–12 years	72	4–7	2,400	60	1.1	15	4,500	1.0	1.4	16	70	400
12–15 years	98	5–1	3,000	75	1.4	15	5,000	1.2	1.8	20	80	400
15–18 years	134	5–8	3,400	85	1.4	15	5,000	1.4	2.0	22	80	400
Girls:												
9–12 years	72	4–7	2,200	55	1.1	15	4,500	0.9	1.3	15	80	400
12–15 years	103	5–2	2,500	62	1.3	15	5,000	1.0	1.5	17	80	400
15–18 years	117	5–4	2,300	58	1.3	15	5,000	0.9	1.3	15	70	400

* Niacin equivalents include dietary sources of the preformed vitamin and the precursor, tryptophan. 60 milligrams tryptophan equals 1 milligram niacin.

statement 28

Calories must be calculated in the diet.

Introduction   The oxidation of food releases heat, when utilized by the human body for the production of energy. Some foodstuffs release more heat than others, and those foods with higher caloric potential must be carefully planned for in the diet. Food scientists have discovered that 1 gram of carbohydrate and 1 gram of protein yield approximately four calories, while 1 gram of fat yields nine calories of energy when metabolized. Most diets consist of carefully measured grams of carbohydrate, protein, and fat.

This statement will allow the student to calculate the number of calories in a variety of foods, and to better understand how the caloric value of foods is derived.

Procedure   1. To calculate calories, use the following and Table 7–7.

Step 1: Determine the food contents of 30 grams of several types of food.

Step 2: Estimate the weight of a "normal" portion of each of the foods in step 1. To calculate the food composition of the "normal" portion divide the weight of the "normal" portion by 30. Next multiply this figure by the food composition values from Step 1.

Step 3: To determine the calories in the "normal" portion of food, multiply the answers in Step 2 by the calories each foodstuff yields (i.e., Carbohydrate 4 cal, Protein 4 cal, and Fat 9 cal).

2. The above chart and steps will provide the number of calories in a selected food based on quantity.
3. The students, after an initial demonstration, should practice calculating a variety of foods.

Teaching Methods   *Performance Objective*

The students should be able to calculate the caloric value of any amount of food based on the method presented.

146

TABLE 7–7. Carbohydrate, Protein and Fat in Basic Food.

Food*	CHO	PRO	FAT
Bread, 1 large slice	15	2.5	0
Biscuits, 4	20	3	2
3% Vegetables†	1	0.5	0
6% Vegetables†	2	0.5	0
20% Vegetables†	6	1	1
Milk (whole)	1.5	1	1
Milk (skim or buttermilk)	1.5	1	0
Egg, 1 medium (50 gm scrambled)	0	6	6
Meat, lean & fish (average value)	0	7	5
Chicken (all poultry and fowl)	0	8	3
Shellfish	0	6	0
Cheese, yellow	0	8	10
Butter or margarine	0	0	25
Butter—5 gm, 1 tsp	0	0	4
Cooked cereal, 180 gm	15	2.5	1
Dry, prepared cereal, 18 gm	15	2.5	1

*Values for 30 grams unless otherwise noted.

†Consult Table 7–8 for list of vegetables in each category.

Adapted from Alexander Marble, Priscilla White, Robert Bradley, and Leo Krall (eds.), *Joslin's Diabetes Mellitus* (11th ed.). Philadelphia: Lea and Febiger, 1971, p. 266.)

Teaching Hints

1. Ask the school dietician or home economics teacher for the "normal" portion of a variety of foods—the more different kinds the better.

2. The following is an example of how to solve the calculations listed under Procedure:

   Assume we decide to calculate the number of calories in a small dish of potato. The potato weighs 120 grams. (30 grams = 1 ounce). Step 1 is to locate on the food scale (Table 7–7) the amount of usable carbohydrate, protein, and fat in 30 grams or 1 ounce. Because potato is considered a 20 percent vegetable (Table 7–8), we find 30 grams of this type of food to be equal to 6 grams of carbohydrate, 1 gram of protein, and no grams of fat. Step 2 is to determine the number of "chart" portions in our sample. Because the table lists the food value for 30 grams and our serving is 120 grams, we must multiply by 4 (120/30). Consequently, in 120 grams of potato we have 24 usable grams of carbohydrate, 4 usable grams of protein, and no fat. In Step 3, we must multiply by the number of calories that 1 gram of usable foodstuff yields. The results from Step 3 are summed to give the total calories in 120 grams of potato.

TABLE 7–8. Classifications of Fruits and Vegetables.

VEGETABLES *Frozen, Fresh, or Canned*		FRUITS *Fresh, Canned (water packed)*		
3 Percent—(Eat Freely)			CHO	
			10 gms	15 gms
Lettuce	Radishes			
Cucumbers, raw	Water Cress			
Spinach	Snap Beans	Grapefruit	150	225
Asparagus	Cauliflower	Strawberries	150	225
Celery	Cabbage	Watermelon	150	225
Mushrooms	Egg Plant	Cantaloupe	150	225
Rhubarb ·	Broccoli	Blackberries	120	180
Sauerkraut	Green Peppers	Orange	100	150
Endive, raw	Kohl Rabi	Pears	90	135
Swiss Chard	Kale	Peaches	90	135
Beet Greens	Summer	Fruit Cocktail	90	135
Dandelions	Squash	Apricots	80	120
		Raspberries	80	120
		Plums	80	120
6 Percent	*20 Percent—*	Pineapple	70	105
Tomatoes	*(Bread Subst)*	Apple	70	105
Turnip	Potatoes	Honeydew Melon	70	105
Carrots	Shell Beans	Blueberries	70	105
Okra	Baked Beans	Cherries	60	90
Pumpkin	Lima Beans	Banana	50	75
Onions	Corn	Prunes (Cooked)	50	75
Squash	Boiled Rice			
Brussels Sprouts	Boiled		*Calorie—Unit of Heat*	
Beets	Macaroni	1 gm CHO	=	4 calories
Green peas		1 gm Protein	=	4 calories
		1 gm fat	=	9 calories

Adapted from Alexander Marble, Priscilla White, Robert Bradley, and Leo Krall (eds.), *Joslin's Diabetes Mellitus* (11th edition). Philadelphia: Lea and Febiger, 1971, pp. 267.

List Food: Potato (120 gm)

	CHO	PRO	FAT
Step 1:	6	1	0
Step 2: $\dfrac{120\,\text{gm}}{30} = 4$	24	4	0
Step 3:	24 gm 4 cal ———— 96 cal	4 gm 4 cal ———— 16 cal	0 gm 9 cal ———— 0

Step 4: Total calories = 112

3. Set up a demonstration showing the number of calories in a variety of foods.

Discussion
1. Which food has the largest number of calories per 150 grams: potato, salad, turkey, whole milk ,skimmed, or nonfat milk?
2. In terms of a weight-reduction diet, what would you have as a midnight snack?

Materials
1. Scales (gram scale is preferred, but any scale can be used).
2. Food scale (Tables 7–7 and 7–8).

statement 29

Diet must be selected to meet individual goals.

Introduction   Each student has determined an energy equilibrium for one day based on the individual intake of food and beverage and the expenditure of energy. Now sufficient information is available to properly plan a diet which will meet the goals of each student regarding weight control. Seven diets are presented in this statement with a caloric range from 1000 to 3000.

Procedure   The students should select an appropriate diet based on their decision to gain or to lose weight according to their desired body weight, percent of body fat, and energy balance.

Teaching Methods   *Performance Objective*

The student should be able to select a diet plan based on the energy balance information from Statement 26 by choosing one of the seven diets provided.

Teaching Hints

1. The student should be able to prepare a profile based upon body composition, diet, and energy expenditure information.

Student	Sex	Weight	% Body Fat	Target % Body Fat	Desired Weight	Energy Expend- iture	Diet Selected	Energy Balance	Time to gain/ lose 1 lb	Time to reach weight desired
Example A	F	145	24	20	139	2200	1500	− 700	5 days	30
Example B	M	125	11	16	131	3500	(3000 + 1000)	+500	7 days	42
Student Profile —	—	—	—	—	—	—	————————	—	—	—

2. Sample calculation:
   From Statement 6, percentage of body fat, target percentage of body fat, and desired weight should have been determined. From State-

150

ment 26, the usual daily caloric intake should have been estimated. Student A weighs 145 lbs. She has a percent of body fat of 24. She decides that 20 percent body fat would be a realistic goal. Using the formula below, pounds overweight can be determined:

$$\text{lbs over/underweight} = \text{Actual Body Wt. (\% Body Fat} - \text{\% Body-Fat Goal)}$$

$$= 145\ (24\%\text{--}20\%)$$

$$= 5.8\ \text{lbs}$$

She decides to lose 6 pounds to a desired actual body weight of 139. From Statement 26 it has been determined that she normally expends about 2200 calories/day. She selects a diet of 1500 calories, thus providing for a negative energy balance of 700 calories.

$$\text{Energy Expenditure (calories/day)} = 2200$$

$$\text{Selected Diet (calories/day)} \quad = 1500$$

The time to lose or gain 1 lb of body fat is determined by the following formula (1 lb of body fat $=$ 3500 calories):

$$\text{Time to Lose/Gain 1 lb of fat} = \frac{3500\ \text{kcal}}{\text{Energy Balance}}$$

$$= \frac{3500}{700}$$

$$= 5\ \text{days}$$

$$\begin{aligned} \text{Time to Reach} \\ \text{Desired Weight} &= \text{Time to Lose/Gain 1 lb of Fat} \times \text{lbs to Reach} \\ & \quad \text{Desired Weight} \end{aligned}$$

$$= 5\ \text{days} \times 6\ \text{lbs}$$

$$= 30\ \text{days}$$

It must be remembered this is only a "rule of thumb" method. Weight gain or weight loss is dependent upon many factors related to the individual.

3. The seven diet plans provided in this statement must be made available to the student completing this lesson.

Discussion   1. Have some selected students discuss the rationale for their diet plans.

2. How does a person accomplish a diet plan? What factors are necessary to adhere to a diet? List the reasons people give for not controlling their energy balance.
3. Are fad diets of any value?

Materials   The seven Eli Lilly Co. diets.

General Rules for All Diets

Measuring Food

Food should be measured. You will need a standard 8-ounce measuring cup and a measuring teaspoon and tablespoon. All measurements are level. Most foods are measured after cooking.

Food Preparation

Meats should be baked, boiled, or broiled. Do not fry foods unless fat allowed in meal is used.

Vegetables may be prepared with the family meals, but your portion should be removed before extra fat or flour is added.

Special Foods

It is not necessary to buy special foods. Select your diet from the same foods purchased for the rest of the family—milk, vegetables, bread, meats, fats, and fruit (fresh, dried, or canned without sugar). "Special dietetic foods" should be thoroughly investigated and usually must be figured in the diet.

Foods to Avoid

Sugar	Pie
Candy	Cake
Honey	Cookies
Jam	Pastries
Jelly	Condensed Milk
Marmalade	Soft Drinks
Syrups	Candy-Coated Gum

Fried, scalloped, or creamed foods
Beer, wine, or other alcoholic beverages

Eat only those foods which are on diet list.

Eat only the amounts of foods on diet.

Do not skip meals.

Do not eat between meals.

The use of the exchange list is based upon the recommendation of the American Diabetes Association and The American Dietetic Association in co-operation with the Diabetes Branch of the U.S. Public Health Service, Department of Health, Education, and Welfare.

TABLE 7–9.   1000 Calorie Diet.

1000 calories (approximately)	carbohydrate	90 Gm.
	protein	60 Gm.
	fat	45 Gm.

Daily menu guide

The foods allowed in your diet should be selected from the seven exchange lists on this page. Menus should be planned on the basis of the menu guide given below. Foods in the same list are interchangeable, because, in the quantities specified, they provide approximately the same amounts of carbohydrate, protein, and fat. For example, when your menu calls for one bread exchange, any item in List 4 may be used in the amount stated. If two bread exchanges are allowed, double the specified amount or use a single exchange of *two* foods in List 4. Sample menus on the reverse side of this sheet illustrate correct use of the exchange lists.

BREAKFAST

1 fruit exchange (List 3)
1 bread exchange (List 4)
2 meat exchanges (List 5)
1/2 milk exchange (List 7)
Coffee or tea (any amount)

LUNCH

2 meat exchanges (List 5)
1 bread exchange (List 4)
Vegetable(s) as desired (List 1)
1 fruit exchange (List 3)
1/2 milk (skimmed) exchange (List 7)
1 fat exchange (List 6)
Coffee or tea (any amount)

DINNER

2 meat exchanges (List 5)
1 bread exchange (List 4)
Vegetable(s) as desired (List 1)
1 vegetable exchange (List 2)
1 fruit exchange (List 3)
1 fat exchange (List 6)
Coffee or tea (any amount)

List 1 allowed as desired
(need not be measured)

Seasonings: Cinnamon, celery salt, garlic, garlic salt, lemon, mustard, mint, nutmeg, parsley, pepper, saccharin and other sugarless sweeteners, spices, vanilla, and vinegar.

Other Foods: Coffee or tea (without sugar or cream), fat-free broth, bouillon, unflavored gelatin, rennet tablets, sour or dill pickles, cranberries (without sugar), rhubarb (without sugar).

Vegetables: Group A—insignificant carbohydrate or calories. You may eat as much as desired of raw vegetable. If cooked vegetable is eaten, limit amount to 1 cup.

Asparagus	Lettuce
Broccoli	Mushrooms
Brussels sprouts	Okra
Cabbage	Peppers, green
Cauliflower	or red
Celery	Radishes
Chicory	Sauerkraut
Cucumbers	String beans
Eggplant	Summer squash
Escarole	Tomatoes
Greens: beet, chard, collard,	Watercress
dandelion, kale, mustard,	
spinach, turnip	

List 2 vegetable exchanges

Each portion supplies approximately 7 Gm. of carbohydrate and 2 Gm. of protein, or 36 calories.

Vegetables: Group B—One serving equals 1/2 cup, or 100 Gm.

Beets	Pumpkin
Carrots	Rutabagas
Onions	Squash, winter
Peas, green	Turnips

TABLE 7–9. (Continued)

List 3 fruit exchanges

(fresh, dried, or canned without sugar)

Each portion supplies approximately 10 Gm. of carbohydrate, or 40 calories.

	household measurement	weight of portion
Apple	1 small (2″ diam.)	80 Gm.
Applesauce	1/2 cup	100 Gm.
Apricots, fresh	2 med	100 Gm.
Apricots, dried	4 halves	20 Gm.
Banana	1/2 small	50 Gm.
Berries	1 cup	150 Gm.
Blueberries	2/3 cup	100 Gm.
Cantaloupe	1/4 (6″ diam.)	200 Gm.
Cherries	10 large	75 Gm.
Dates	2	15 Gm.
Figs, fresh	2 large	50 Gm.
Figs, dried	1 small	15 Gm.
Grapefruit	1/2 small	125 Gm.
Grapefruit juice	1/2 cup	100 Gm.
Grapes	12	75 Gm.
Grape juice	1/4 cup	60 Gm.
Honeydew melon	1/8 (7″)	150 Gm.
Mango	1/2 small	70 Gm.
Orange	1 small	100 Gm.
Orange juice	1/2 cup	100 Gm.
Papaya	1/3 med	100 Gm.
Peach	1 med	100 Gm.
Pear	1 small	100 Gm.
Pineapple	1/2 cup	80 Gm.
Pineapple juice	1/3 cup	80 Gm.
Plums	2 med	100 Gm.
Prunes, dried	2	25 Gm.
Raisins	2 tbsp	15 Gm.
Tangerine	1 large	100 Gm.
Watermelon	1 cup	175 Gm.

List 4 bread exchanges

Each portion supplies approximately 15 Gm. of carbohydrate and 2 Gm. of protein, or 68 calories.

	household measurement	weight of portion
Bread	1 slice	25 Gm.
Biscuit, roll	1 (2″ diam.)	35 Gm.
Muffin	1 (2″ diam.)	35 Gm.
Cornbread	1 1/2″ cube	35 Gm.
Flour	2 1/2 tbsp	20 Gm.
Cereal, cooked	1/2 cup	100 Gm.
Cereal, dry (flakes or puffed)	3/4 cup	20 Gm.
Rice or grits, cooked	1/2 cup	100 Gm.
Spaghetti, noodles, etc.	1/2 cup	100 Gm.
Crackers, graham	2	20 Gm.
Crackers, oyster	20 (1/2 cup)	20 Gm.
Crackers, saltine	5	20 Gm.
Crackers, soda	3	20 Gm.
Crackers, round	6-8	20 Gm.
Vegetables		
Beans (Lima, navy, etc.), dry, cooked	1/2 cup	90 Gm.
Peas (split peas, etc.), dry, cooked	1/2 cup	90 Gm.
Baked beans, no pork	1/4 cup	50 Gm.
Corn	1/3 cup	80 Gm.
Parsnips	2/3 cup	125 Gm.
Potato, white, baked or boiled	1 (2″ diam.)	100 Gm.
Potatoes, white, mashed	1/2 cup	100 Gm.
Potatoes, sweet, or yams	1/4 cup	50 Gm.
Sponge cake, plain	1 1/2″ cube	25 Gm.
Ice cream (Omit 2 fat exchanges)	1/2 cup	70 Gm.

List 5 meat exchanges

Each portion supplies approximately 7 Gm. of protein and 5 Gm. of fat, or 73 calories. (30 Gm. equal 1 oz.)

	household measurement	weight of portion
Meat and poultry (beef, lamb, pork, liver, chicken, etc.) (med. fat)	1 slice (3″ x 2″ x 1/8″)	30 Gm.
Cold cuts	1 slice (4 1/2″ sq., 1/8″ thick)	45 Gm.
Frankfurter	1 (8-9 per lb.)	50 Gm.
Codfish, mackerel, etc.	1 slice (2″ x 2″ x 1″)	30 Gm.
Salmon, tuna, crab	1/4 cup	30 Gm.
Oysters, shrimp, clams	5 small	45 Gm.
Sardines	3 med	30 Gm.
Cheese, cheddar, American	1 slice (3 1/2″ x 1 1/2″ x 1/4″)	30 Gm.
Cheese, cottage	1/4 cup	45 Gm.
Egg	1	50 Gm.
Peanut butter	2 tbsp	30 Gm.

Limit peanut butter to one exchange per day unless allowance is made for carbohydrate in the diet plan.

List 6 fat exchanges

Each portion supplies approximately 5 Gm. of fat, or 45 calories.

	household measurement	weight of portion
Butter or margarine	1 tsp	5 Gm.
Bacon, crisp	1 slice	10 Gm.
Cream, light	2 tbsp	30 Gm.
Cream, heavy	1 tbsp	15 Gm.
Cream cheese	1 tbsp	15 Gm.
French dressing	1 tbsp	15 Gm.
Mayonnaise	1 tsp	5 Gm.
Oil or cooking fat	1 tsp	5 Gm.
Nuts	6 small	10 Gm.
Olives	5 small	50 Gm.
Avocado	1/8 (4″ diam.)	25 Gm.

List 7 milk exchanges

Each portion supplies approximately 12 Gm. of carbohydrate, 8 Gm. of protein, and 10 Gm. of fat, or 170 calories.

	household measurement	weight of portion
Milk, whole	1 cup	240 Gm.
Milk, evaporated	1/2 cup	120 Gm.
*Milk, powdered	1/4 cup	35 Gm.
*Buttermilk	1 cup	240 Gm.

*Add 2 fat exchanges if milk is fat-free.

TABLE 7–10. 1200 Calorie Diet.

1200 calories

(approximately)

	carbohydrate	125 Gm.
	protein	60 Gm.
	fat	50 Gm.

Daily menu guide

The foods allowed in your diet should be selected from the seven exchange lists on this page. Menus should be planned on the basis of the menu guide given below. Foods in the same list are interchangeable, because, in the quantities specified, they provide approximately the same amounts of carbohydrate, protein, and fat. For example, when your menu calls for one bread exchange, any item in List 4 may be used in the amount stated. If two bread exchanges are allowed, double the specified amount or use a single exchange of *two* foods in List 4. Sample menus on the reverse side of this sheet illustrate correct use of the exchange lists.

BREAKFAST

1 fruit exchange (List 3)
1 bread exchange (List 4)
1 meat exchange (List 5)
1 milk exchange (List 7)
Coffee or tea (any amount)

LUNCH

2 meat exchanges (List 5)
1 1/2 bread exchanges (List 4)
Vegetable(s) as desired (List 1)
1 fruit exchange (List 3)
1 milk (skimmed) exchange (List 7)
2 fat exchanges (List 6)
Coffee or tea (any amount)

DINNER

2 meat exchanges (List 5)
1 1/2 bread exchanges (List 4)
Vegetable(s) as desired (List 1)
1 vegetable exchange (List 2)
1 fruit exchange (List 3)
1 fat exchange (List 6)
Coffee or tea (any amount)

List 1 allowed as desired

(need not be measured)

Seasonings: Cinnamon, celery salt, garlic, garlic salt, lemon, mustard, mint, nutmeg, parsley, pepper, saccharin and other sugarless sweeteners, spices, vanilla, and vinegar.

Other Foods: Coffee or tea (without sugar or cream), fat-free broth, bouillon, unflavored gelatin, rennet tablets, sour or dill pickles, cranberries (without sugar), rhubarb (without sugar).

Vegetables: Group A—insignificant carbohydrate or calories. You may eat as much as desired of raw vegetable. If cooked vegetable is eaten, limit amount to 1 cup.

Asparagus	Lettuce
Broccoli	Mushrooms
Brussels sprouts	Okra
Cabbage	Peppers, green
Cauliflower	or red
Celery	Radishes
Chicory	Sauerkraut
Cucumbers	String beans
Eggplant	Summer squash
Escarole	Tomatoes
Greens: beet, chard, collard,	Watercress
dandelion, kale, mustard,	
spinach, turnip	

List 2 vegetable exchanges

Each portion supplies approximately 7 Gm. of carbohydrate and 2 Gm. of protein, or 36 calories.

Vegetables: Group B—One serving equals 1/2 cup, or 100 Gm.

Beets	Pumpkin
Carrots	Rutabagas
Onions	Squash, winter
Peas, green	Turnips

TABLE 7–10. (Continued)

List 3 fruit exchanges
(fresh, dried, or canned without sugar)

Each portion supplies approximately 10 Gm. of carbohydrate, or 40 calories.

	household measurement	weight of portion
Apple	1 small (2″ diam.)	80 Gm.
Applesauce	1/2 cup	100 Gm.
Apricots, fresh	2 med.	100 Gm.
Apricots, dried	4 halves	20 Gm.
Banana	1/2 small	50 Gm.
Berries	1 cup	150 Gm.
Blueberries	2/3 cup	100 Gm.
Cantaloupe	1/4 (6″ diam.)	200 Gm.
Cherries	10 large	75 Gm.
Dates	2	15 Gm.
Figs, fresh	2 large	50 Gm.
Figs, dried	1 small	15 Gm.
Grapefruit	1/2 small	125 Gm.
Grapefruit juice	1/2 cup	100 Gm.
Grapes	12	75 Gm.
Grape juice	1/4 cup	60 Gm.
Honeydew melon	1/8 (7″)	150 Gm.
Mango	1/2 small	70 Gm.
Orange	1 small	100 Gm.
Orange juice	1/2 cup	100 Gm.
Papaya	1/3 med.	100 Gm.
Peach	1 med.	100 Gm.
Pear	1 small	100 Gm.
Pineapple	1/2 cup	80 Gm.
Pineapple juice	1/3 cup	80 Gm.
Plums	2 med.	100 Gm.
Prunes, dried	2	25 Gm.
Raisins	2 tbsp.	15 Gm.
Tangerine	1 large	100 Gm.
Watermelon	1 cup	175 Gm.

List 4 bread exchanges

Each portion supplies approximately 15 Gm. of carbohydrate and 2 Gm. of protein, or 68 calories.

	household measurement	weight of portion
Bread	1 slice	25 Gm.
Biscuit, roll	1 (2″ diam.)	35 Gm.
Muffin	1 (2″ diam.)	35 Gm.
Cornbread	1 1/2″ cube	35 Gm.
Flour	2 1/2 tbsp.	20 Gm.
Cereal, cooked	1/2 cup	100 Gm.
Cereal, dry (flakes or puffed)	3/4 cup	20 Gm.
Rice or grits, cooked	1/2 cup	100 Gm.
Spaghetti, noodles, etc.	1/2 cup	100 Gm.
Crackers, graham	2	20 Gm.
Crackers, oyster	20 (1/2 cup)	20 Gm.
Crackers, saltine	5	20 Gm.
Crackers, soda	3	20 Gm.
Crackers, round	6-8	20 Gm.
Vegetables		
Beans (Lima, navy, etc.), dry, cooked	1/2 cup	90 Gm.
Peas (split peas, etc.), dry, cooked	1/2 cup	90 Gm.
Baked beans, no pork	1/4 cup	50 Gm.
Corn	1/3 cup	80 Gm.
Parsnips	2/3 cup	125 Gm.
Potato, white, baked or boiled	1 (2″ diam.)	100 Gm.
Potatoes, white, mashed	1/2 cup	100 Gm.
Potatoes, sweet, or yams	1/4 cup	50 Gm.
Sponge cake, plain	1 1/2″ cube	25 Gm.
Ice cream (Omit 2 fat exchanges)	1/2 cup	70 Gm.

List 5 meat exchanges

Each portion supplies approximately 7 Gm. of protein and 5 Gm. of fat, or 73 calories. (30 Gm. equal 1 oz.)

	household measurement	weight of portion
Meat and poultry (beef, lamb, pork, liver, chicken, etc.) (med. fat)	1 slice (3″ x 2″ x 1/8″)	30 Gm.
Cold cuts	1 slice (4 1/2″ sq., 1/8″ thick)	45 Gm.
Frankfurter	1 (8-9 per lb.)	50 Gm.
Codfish, mackerel, etc.	1 slice (2″ x 2″ x 1″)	30 Gm.
Salmon, tuna, crab	1/4 cup	30 Gm.
Oysters, shrimp, clams	5 small	45 Gm.
Sardines	3 med.	30 Gm.
Cheese, cheddar, American	1 slice (3 1/2″ x 1 1/2″ x 1/4″)	30 Gm.
Cheese, cottage	1/4 cup	45 Gm.
Egg	1	50 Gm.
Peanut butter	2 tbsp.	30 Gm.

Limit peanut butter to one exchange per day unless allowance is made for carbohydrate in the diet plan.

List 6 fat exchanges

Each portion supplies approximately 5 Gm. of fat, or 45 calories.

	household measurement	weight of portion
Butter or margarine	1 tsp.	5 Gm.
Bacon, crisp	1 slice	10 Gm.
Cream, light	2 tbsp.	30 Gm.
Cream, heavy	1 tbsp.	15 Gm.
Cream cheese	1 tbsp.	15 Gm.
French dressing	1 tbsp.	15 Gm.
Mayonnaise	1 tsp.	5 Gm.
Oil or cooking fat	1 tsp.	5 Gm.
Nuts	6 small	10 Gm.
Olives	5 small	50 Gm.
Avocado	1/8 (4″ diam.)	25 Gm.

List 7 milk exchanges

Each portion supplies approximately 12 Gm. of carbohydrate, 8 Gm. of protein, and 10 Gm. of fat, or 170 calories.

	household measurement	weight of portion
Milk, whole	1 cup	240 Gm.
Milk, evaporated	1/2 cup	120 Gm.
*Milk, powdered	1/4 cup	35 Gm.
*Buttermilk	1 cup	240 Gm.

*Add 2 fat exchanges if milk is fat-free.

TABLE 7–11. 1500 Calorie Diet.

1500 calories { carbohydrate 150 Gm.
(approximately) protein 70 Gm.
fat 70 Gm.

Daily menu guide

The foods allowed in your diet should be selected from the seven exchange lists on this page. Menus should be planned on the basis of the menu guide given below. Foods in the same list are interchangeable, because, in the quantities specified, they provide approximately the same amounts of carbohydrate, protein, and fat. For example, when your menu calls for one bread exchange, any item in List 4 may be used in the amount stated. If two bread exchanges are allowed, double the specified amount or use a single exchange of *two* foods in List 4. Sample menus on the reverse side of this sheet illustrate correct use of the exchange lists.

BREAKFAST

1 fruit exchange (List 3)
2 bread exchanges (List 4)
1 meat exchange (List 5)
1 milk exchange (List 7)
2 fat exchanges (List 6)
Coffee or tea (any amount)

LUNCH

2 meat exchanges (List 5)
2 bread exchanges (List 4)
Vegetable(s) as desired (List 1)
1 fruit exchange (List 3)
1 milk exchange (List 7)
1 fat exchange (List 6)
Coffee or tea (any amount)

DINNER

2 meat exchanges (List 5)
1 1/2 bread exchanges (List 4)
Vegetable(s) as desired (List 1)
1 vegetable exchange (List 2)
1 fruit exchange (List 3)
1/2 milk exchange (List 7)
1 fat exchange (List 6)
Coffee or tea (any amount)

List 1 allowed as desired

(need not be measured)

Seasonings: Cinnamon, celery salt, garlic, garlic salt, lemon, mustard, mint, nutmeg, parsley, pepper, saccharin and other sugarless sweeteners, spices, vanilla, and vinegar.

Other Foods: Coffee or tea (without sugar or cream), fat-free broth, bouillon, unflavored gelatin, rennet tablets, sour or dill pickles, cranberries (without sugar), rhubarb (without sugar).

Vegetables: Group A—insignificant carbohydrate or calories. You may eat as much as desired of raw vegetable. If cooked vegetable is eaten, limit amount to 1 cup.

Asparagus	Lettuce
Broccoli	Mushrooms
Brussels sprouts	Okra
Cabbage	Peppers, green
Cauliflower	or red
Celery	Radishes
Chicory	Sauerkraut
Cucumbers	String beans
Eggplant	Summer squash
Escarole	Tomatoes
Greens: beet, chard, collard,	Watercress
dandelion, kale, mustard,	
spinach, turnip	

List 2 vegetable exchanges

Each portion supplies approximately 7 Gm. of carbohydrate and 2 Gm. of protein, or 36 calories.

Vegetables: Group B—One serving equals 1/2 cup, or 100 Gm.

Beets	Pumpkin
Carrots	Rutabagas
Onions	Squash, winter
Peas, green	Turnips

By permission of E. Lilly and Company, Indianapolis. Indiana.

TABLE 7–11. (Continued)

List 3 fruit exchanges

(fresh, dried, or canned without sugar)

Each portion supplies approximately 10 Gm. of carbohydrate, or 40 calories.

	household measurement	weight of portion
Apple	1 small (2″ diam.)	80 Gm.
Applesauce	1/2 cup	100 Gm.
Apricots, fresh	2 med	100 Gm.
Apricots, dried	4 halves	20 Gm.
Banana	1/2 small	50 Gm.
Berries	1 cup	150 Gm.
Blueberries	2/3 cup	100 Gm.
Cantaloupe	1/4 (6″ diam.)	200 Gm.
Cherries	10 large	75 Gm.
Dates	2	15 Gm.
Figs, fresh	2 large	50 Gm.
Figs, dried	1 small	15 Gm.
Grapefruit	1/2 small	125 Gm.
Grapefruit juice	1/2 cup	100 Gm.
Grapes	12	75 Gm.
Grape juice	1/4 cup	60 Gm.
Honeydew melon	1/8 (7″)	150 Gm.
Mango	1/2 small	70 Gm.
Orange	1 small	100 Gm.
Orange juice	1/2 cup	100 Gm.
Papaya	1/3 med	100 Gm.
Peach	1 med	100 Gm.
Pear	1 small	100 Gm.
Pineapple	1/2 cup	80 Gm.
Pineapple juice	1/3 cup	80 Gm.
Plums	2 med	100 Gm.
Prunes, dried	2	25 Gm.
Raisins	2 tbsp	15 Gm.
Tangerine	1 large	100 Gm.
Watermelon	1 cup	175 Gm.

List 4 bread exchanges

Each portion supplies approximately 15 Gm. of carbohydrate and 2 Gm. of protein, or 68 calories.

	household measurement	weight of portion
Bread	1 slice	25 Gm.
Biscuit, roll	1 (2″ diam.)	35 Gm.
Muffin	1 (2″ diam.)	35 Gm.
Cornbread	1 1/2″ cube	35 Gm.
Flour	2 1/2 tbsp	20 Gm.
Cereal, cooked	1/2 cup	100 Gm.
Cereal, dry (flakes or puffed)	3/4 cup	20 Gm.
Rice or grits, cooked	1/2 cup	100 Gm.
Spaghetti, noodles, etc.	1/2 cup	100 Gm.
Crackers, graham	2	20 Gm.
Crackers, oyster	20 (1/2 cup)	20 Gm.
Crackers, saltine	5	20 Gm.
Crackers, soda	3	20 Gm.
Crackers, round	6-8	20 Gm.
Vegetables		
Beans (Lima, navy, etc.), dry, cooked	1/2 cup	90 Gm.
Peas (split peas, etc.), dry, cooked	1/2 cup	90 Gm.
Baked beans, no pork	1/4 cup	50 Gm.
Corn	1/3 cup	80 Gm.
Parsnips	2/3 cup	125 Gm.
Potato, white, baked or boiled	1 (2″ diam.)	100 Gm.
Potatoes, white, mashed	1/2 cup	100 Gm.
Potatoes, sweet, or yams	1/4 cup	50 Gm.
Sponge cake, plain	1 1/2″ cube	25 Gm.
Ice cream (Omit 2 fat exchanges)	1/2 cup	70 Gm.

List 5 meat exchanges

Each portion supplies approximately 7 Gm. of protein and 5 Gm. of fat, or 73 calories. (30 Gm. equal 1 oz.)

	household measurement	weight of portion
Meat and poultry (beef, lamb, pork, liver, chicken, etc.) (med. fat)	1 slice (3″ x 2″ x 1/8″)	30 Gm.
Cold cuts	1 slice (4 1/2″ sq., 1/8″ thick)	45 Gm.
Frankfurter	1 (8-9 per lb.)	50 Gm.
Codfish, mackerel, etc.	1 slice (2″ x 2″ x 1″)	30 Gm.
Salmon, tuna, crab	1/4 cup	30 Gm.
Oysters, shrimp, clams	5 small	45 Gm.
Sardines	3 med	30 Gm.
Cheese, cheddar, American	1 slice (3 1/2″ x 1 1/2″ x 1/4″)	30 Gm.
Cheese, cottage	1/4 cup	45 Gm.
Egg	1	50 Gm.
Peanut butter	2 tbsp	30 Gm.

Limit peanut butter to one exchange per day unless allowance is made for carbohydrate in the diet plan.

List 6 fat exchanges

Each portion supplies approximately 5 Gm. of fat, or 45 calories.

	household measurement	weight of portion
Butter or margarine	1 tsp	5 Gm.
Bacon, crisp	1 slice	10 Gm.
Cream, light	2 tbsp	30 Gm.
Cream, heavy	1 tbsp	15 Gm.
Cream cheese	1 tbsp	15 Gm.
French dressing	1 tbsp	15 Gm.
Mayonnaise	1 tsp	5 Gm.
Oil or cooking fat	1 tsp	5 Gm.
Nuts	6 small	10 Gm.
Olives	5 small	50 Gm.
Avocado	1/8 (4″ diam.)	25 Gm.

List 7 milk exchanges

Each portion supplies approximately 12 Gm. of carbohydrate, 8 Gm. of protein, and 10 Gm. of fat, or 170 calories.

	household measurement	weight of portion
Milk, whole	1 cup	240 Gm.
Milk, evaporated	1/2 cup	120 Gm.
*Milk, powdered	1/4 cup	35 Gm.
*Buttermilk	1 cup	240 Gm.

*Add 2 fat exchanges if milk is fat-free.

TABLE 7–12. 2000 Calorie Diet.

2000 calories (approximately)	carbohydrate	210 Gm.
	protein	90 Gm.
	fat	90 Gm.

Daily menu guide

The foods allowed in your diet should be selected from the seven exchange lists on this page. Menus should be planned on the basis of the menu guide given below. Foods in the same list are interchangeable, because, in the quantities specified, they provide approximately the same amounts of carbohydrate, protein, and fat. For example, when your menu calls for one bread exchange, any item in List 4 may be used in the amount stated. If two bread exchanges are allowed, double the specified amount or use a single exchange of *two* foods in List 4. Sample menus on the reverse side of this sheet illustrate correct use of the exchange lists.

BREAKFAST

1 fruit exchange (List 3)
3 bread exchanges (List 4)
2 meat exchanges (List 5)
1 milk exchange (List 7)
2 fat exchanges (List 6)
Coffee or tea (any amount)

LUNCH

2 meat exchanges (List 5)
2 bread exchanges (List 4)
Vegetable(s) as desired (List 1)
1 vegetable exchange (List 2)
2 fruit exchanges (List 3)
1 milk exchange (List 7)
2 fat exchanges (List 6)
Coffee or tea (any amount)

DINNER

3 meat exchanges (List 5)
2 bread exchanges (List 4)
Vegetable(s) as desired (List 1)
1 vegetable exchange (List 2)
2 fruit exchanges (List 3)
1 milk exchange (List 7)
2 fat exchanges (List 6)
Coffee or tea (any amount)

List 1 allowed as desired

(need not be measured)

Seasonings: Cinnamon, celery salt, garlic, garlic salt, lemon, mustard, mint, nutmeg, parsley, pepper, saccharin and other sugarless sweeteners, spices, vanilla, and vinegar.

Other Foods: Coffee or tea (without sugar or cream), fat-free broth, bouillon, unflavored gelatin, rennet tablets, sour or dill pickles, cranberries (without sugar), rhubarb (without sugar).

Vegetables: Group A—insignificant carbohydrate or calories. You may eat as much as desired of raw vegetable. If cooked vegetable is eaten, limit amount to 1 cup.

Asparagus	Lettuce
Broccoli	Mushrooms
Brussels sprouts	Okra
Cabbage	Peppers, green
Cauliflower	or red
Celery	Radishes
Chicory	Sauerkraut
Cucumbers	String beans
Eggplant	Summer squash
Escarole	Tomatoes
Greens: beet, chard, collard,	Watercress
dandelion, kale, mustard,	
spinach, turnip	

List 2 vegetable exchanges

Each portion supplies approximately 7 Gm. of carbohydrate and 2 Gm. of protein, or 36 calories.

Vegetables: Group B—One serving equals 1/2 cup, or 100 Gm.

Beets	Pumpkin
Carrots	Rutabagas
Onions	Squash, winter
Peas, green	Turnips

TABLE 7–12. (Continued)

List 3 fruit exchanges

(fresh, dried, or canned without sugar)

Each portion supplies approximately 10 Gm. of carbohydrate, or 40 calories.

	household measurement	weight of portion
Apple	1 small (2″ diam.)	80 Gm.
Applesauce	1/2 cup	100 Gm.
Apricots, fresh	2 med.	100 Gm.
Apricots, dried	4 halves	20 Gm.
Banana	1/2 small	50 Gm.
Berries	1 cup	150 Gm.
Blueberries	2/3 cup	100 Gm.
Cantaloupe	1/4 (6″ diam.)	200 Gm.
Cherries	10 large	75 Gm.
Dates	2	15 Gm.
Figs, fresh	2 large	50 Gm.
Figs, dried	1 small	15 Gm.
Grapefruit	1/2 small	125 Gm.
Grapefruit juice	1/2 cup	100 Gm.
Grapes	12	75 Gm.
Grape juice	1/4 cup	60 Gm.
Honeydew melon	1/8 (7″)	150 Gm.
Mango	1/2 small	70 Gm.
Orange	1 small	100 Gm.
Orange juice	1/2 cup	100 Gm.
Papaya	1/3 med.	100 Gm.
Peach	1 med.	100 Gm.
Pear	1 small	100 Gm.
Pineapple	1/2 cup	80 Gm.
Pineapple juice	1/3 cup	80 Gm.
Plums	2 med.	100 Gm.
Prunes, dried	2	25 Gm.
Raisins	2 tbsp.	15 Gm.
Tangerine	1 large	100 Gm.
Watermelon	1 cup	175 Gm.

List 4 bread exchanges

Each portion supplies approximately 15 Gm. of carbohydrate and 2 Gm. of protein, or 68 calories.

	household measurement	weight of portion
Bread	1 slice	25 Gm.
Biscuit, roll	1 (2″ diam.)	35 Gm.
Muffin	1 (2″ diam.)	35 Gm.
Cornbread	1 1/2″ cube	35 Gm.
Flour	2 1/2 tbsp.	20 Gm.
Cereal, cooked	1/2 cup	100 Gm.
Cereal, dry (flakes or puffed)	3/4 cup	20 Gm.
Rice or grits, cooked	1/2 cup	100 Gm.
Spaghetti, noodles, etc.	1/2 cup	100 Gm.
Crackers, graham	2	20 Gm.
Crackers, oyster	20 (1/2 cup)	20 Gm.
Crackers, saltine	5	20 Gm.
Crackers, soda	3	20 Gm.
Crackers, round	6-8	20 Gm.
Vegetables		
Beans (Lima, navy, etc.), dry, cooked	1/2 cup	90 Gm.
Peas (split peas, etc.), dry, cooked	1/2 cup	90 Gm.
Baked beans, no pork	1/4 cup	50 Gm.
Corn	1/3 cup	80 Gm.
Parsnips	2/3 cup	125 Gm.
Potato, white, baked or boiled	1 (2″ diam.)	100 Gm.
Potatoes, white, mashed	1/2 cup	100 Gm.
Potatoes, sweet, or yams	1/4 cup	50 Gm.
Sponge cake, plain	1 1/2″ cube	25 Gm.
Ice cream (Omit 2 fat exchanges)	1/2 cup	70 Gm.

List 5 meat exchanges

Each portion supplies approximately 7 Gm. of protein and 5 Gm. of fat, or 73 calories. (30 Gm. equal 1 oz.)

	household measurement	weight of portion
Meat and poultry (beef, lamb, pork, liver, chicken, etc.) (med. fat)	1 slice (3″ x 2″ x 1/8″)	30 Gm.
Cold cuts	1 slice (4 1/2″ sq., 1/8″ thick)	45 Gm.
Frankfurter	1 (8-9 per lb.)	50 Gm.
Codfish, mackerel, etc.	1 slice (2″ x 2″ x 1″)	30 Gm.
Salmon, tuna, crab	1/4 cup	30 Gm.
Oysters, shrimp, clams	5 small	45 Gm.
Sardines	3 med.	30 Gm.
Cheese, cheddar, American	1 slice (3 1/2″ x 1 1/2″ x 1/4″)	30 Gm.
Cheese, cottage	1/4 cup	45 Gm.
Egg	1	50 Gm.
Peanut butter	2 tbsp.	30 Gm.

Limit peanut butter to one exchange per day unless allowance is made for carbohydrate in the diet plan.

List 6 fat exchanges

Each portion supplies approximately 5 Gm. of fat, or 45 calories.

	household measurement	weight of portion
Butter or margarine	1 tsp.	5 Gm.
Bacon, crisp	1 slice	10 Gm.
Cream, light	2 tbsp.	30 Gm.
Cream, heavy	1 tbsp.	15 Gm.
Cream cheese	1 tbsp.	15 Gm.
French dressing	1 tbsp.	15 Gm.
Mayonnaise	1 tsp.	5 Gm.
Oil or cooking fat	1 tsp.	5 Gm.
Nuts	6 small	10 Gm.
Olives	5 small	50 Gm.
Avocado	1/8 (4″ diam.)	25 Gm.

List 7 milk exchanges

Each portion supplies approximately 12 Gm. of carbohydrate, 8 Gm. of protein, and 10 Gm. of fat, or 170 calories.

	household measurement	weight of portion
Milk, whole	1 cup	240 Gm.
Milk, evaporated	1/2 cup	120 Gm.
*Milk, powdered	1/4 cup	35 Gm.
*Buttermilk	1 cup	240 Gm.

*Add 2 fat exchanges if milk is fat-free.

TABLE 7–13. 2200 Calorie Diet.

2200 calories
(approximately)

carbohydrate	250 Gm.
protein	90 Gm.
fat	90 Gm.

Daily menu guide

The foods allowed in your diet should be selected from the seven exchange lists on this page. Menus should be planned on the basis of the menu guide given below. Foods in the same list are interchangeable, because, in the quantities specified, they provide approximately the same amounts of carbohydrate, protein, and fat. For example, when your menu calls for one bread exchange, any item in List 4 may be used in the amount stated. If two bread exchanges are allowed, double the specified amount or use a single exchange of *two* foods in List 4. Sample menus on the reverse side of this sheet illustrate correct use of the exchange lists.

BREAKFAST

2 fruit exchanges (List 3)
3 1/2 bread exchanges (List 4)
2 meat exchanges (List 5)
1 milk exchange (List 7)
2 fat exchanges (List 6)
Coffee or tea (any amount)

LUNCH

2 meat exchanges (List 5)
4 bread exchanges (List 4)
Vegetable(s) as desired (List 1)
1 fruit exchange (List 3)
1 milk exchange (List 7)
2 fat exchanges (List 6)
Coffee or tea (any amount)

DINNER

2 meat exchanges (List 5)
3 bread exchanges (List 4)
Vegetable(s) as desired (List 1)
1 vegetable exchange (List 2)
2 fruit exchanges (List 3)
1 milk exchange (List 7)
2 fat exchanges (List 6)
Coffee or tea (any amount)

List 1 allowed as desired
(need not be measured)

Seasonings: Cinnamon, celery salt, garlic, garlic salt, lemon, mustard, mint, nutmeg, parsley, pepper, saccharin and other sugarless sweeteners, spices, vanilla, and vinegar.

Other Foods: Coffee or tea (without sugar or cream), fat-free broth, bouillon, unflavored gelatin, rennet tablets, sour or dill pickles, cranberries (without sugar), rhubarb (without sugar).

Vegetables: Group A—insignificant carbohydrate or calories. You may eat as much as desired of raw vegetable. If cooked vegetable is eaten, limit amount to 1 cup.

Asparagus	Lettuce
Broccoli	Mushrooms
Brussels sprouts	Okra
Cabbage	Peppers, green
Cauliflower	or red
Celery	Radishes
Chicory	Sauerkraut
Cucumbers	String beans
Eggplant	Summer squash
Escarole	Tomatoes
Greens: beet, chard, collard,	Watercress
dandelion, kale, mustard,	
spinach, turnip	

List 2 vegetable exchanges

Each portion supplies approximately 7 Gm. of carbohydrate and 2 Gm. of protein, or 36 calories.

Vegetables: Group B—One serving equals 1/2 cup, or 100 Gm.

Beets	Pumpkin
Carrots	Rutabagas
Onions	Squash, winter
Peas, green	Turnips

TABLE 7–13. (Continued)

List 3 fruit exchanges

(fresh, dried, or canned without sugar)

Each portion supplies approximately 10 Gm. of carbohydrate, or 40 calories.

	household measurement	weight of portion
Apple	1 small (2″ diam.)	80 Gm.
Applesauce	1/2 cup	100 Gm.
Apricots, fresh	2 med.	100 Gm.
Apricots, dried	4 halves	20 Gm.
Banana	1/2 small	50 Gm.
Berries	1 cup	150 Gm.
Blueberries	2/3 cup	100 Gm.
Cantaloupe	1/4 (6″ diam.)	200 Gm.
Cherries	10 large	75 Gm.
Dates	2	15 Gm.
Figs, fresh	2 large	50 Gm.
Figs, dried	1 small	15 Gm.
Grapefruit	1/2 small	125 Gm.
Grapefruit juice	1/2 cup	100 Gm.
Grapes	12	75 Gm.
Grape juice	1/4 cup	60 Gm.
Honeydew melon	1/8 (7″)	150 Gm.
Mango	1/2 small	70 Gm.
Orange	1 small	100 Gm.
Orange juice	1/2 cup	100 Gm.
Papaya	1/3 med.	100 Gm.
Peach	1 med.	100 Gm.
Pear	1 small	100 Gm.
Pineapple	1/2 cup	80 Gm.
Pineapple juice	1/3 cup	80 Gm.
Plums	2 med.	100 Gm.
Prunes, dried	2	25 Gm.
Raisins	2 tbsp.	15 Gm.
Tangerine	1 large	100 Gm.
Watermelon	1 cup	175 Gm.

List 4 bread exchanges

Each portion supplies approximately 15 Gm. of carbohydrate and 2 Gm. of protein, or 68 calories.

	household measurement	weight of portion
Bread	1 slice	25 Gm.
Biscuit, roll	1 (2″ diam.)	35 Gm.
Muffin	1 (2″ diam.)	35 Gm.
Cornbread	1 1/2″ cube	35 Gm.
Flour	2 1/2 tbsp.	20 Gm.
Cereal, cooked	1/2 cup	100 Gm.
Cereal, dry (flakes or puffed)	3/4 cup	20 Gm.
Rice or grits, cooked	1/2 cup	100 Gm.
Spaghetti, noodles, etc.	1/2 cup	100 Gm.
Crackers, graham	2	20 Gm.
Crackers, oyster	20 (1/2 cup)	20 Gm.
Crackers, saltine	5	20 Gm.
Crackers, soda	3	20 Gm.
Crackers, round	6-8	20 Gm.
Vegetables		
Beans (Lima, navy, etc.), dry, cooked	1/2 cup	90 Gm.
Peas (split peas, etc.), dry, cooked	1/2 cup	90 Gm.
Baked beans, no pork	1/4 cup	50 Gm.
Corn	1/3 cup	80 Gm.
Parsnips	2/3 cup	125 Gm.
Potato, white, baked or boiled	1 (2″ diam.)	100 Gm.
Potatoes, white, mashed	1/2 cup	100 Gm.
Potatoes, sweet, or yams	1/4 cup	50 Gm.
Sponge cake, plain	1 1/2″ cube	25 Gm.
Ice cream (Omit 2 fat exchanges)	1/2 cup	70 Gm.

List 5 meat exchanges

Each portion supplies approximately 7 Gm. of protein and 5 Gm. of fat, or 73 calories. (30 Gm. equal 1 oz.)

	household measurement	weight of portion
Meat and poultry (beef, lamb, pork, liver, chicken, etc.) (med. fat)	1 slice (3″ x 2″ x 1/8″)	30 Gm.
Cold cuts	1 slice (4 1/2″ sq., 1/8″ thick)	45 Gm.
Frankfurter	1 (8-9 per lb.)	50 Gm.
Codfish, mackerel, etc.	1 slice (2″ x 2″ x 1″)	30 Gm.
Salmon, tuna, crab	1/4 cup	30 Gm.
Oysters, shrimp, clams	5 small	45 Gm.
Sardines	3 med.	30 Gm.
Cheese, cheddar, American	1 slice (3 1/2″ x 1 1/2″ x 1/4″)	30 Gm.
Cheese, cottage	1/4 cup	45 Gm.
Egg	1	50 Gm.
Peanut butter	2 tbsp.	30 Gm.

Limit peanut butter to one exchange per day unless allowance is made for carbohydrate in the diet plan.

List 6 fat exchanges

Each portion supplies approximately 5 Gm. of fat, or 45 calories.

	household measurement	weight of portion
Butter or margarine	1 tsp.	5 Gm.
Bacon	1 slice	10 Gm.
Cream, light	2 tbsp.	30 Gm.
Cream, heavy	1 tbsp.	15 Gm.
Cream cheese	1 tbsp.	15 Gm.
French dressing	1 tbsp.	15 Gm.
Mayonnaise	1 tsp.	5 Gm.
Oil or cooking fat	1 tsp.	5 Gm.
Nuts	6 small	10 Gm.
Olives	5 small	50 Gm.
Avocado	1/8 (4″ diam.)	25 Gm.

List 7 milk exchanges

Each portion supplies approximately 12 Gm. of carbohydrate, 8 Gm. of protein, and 10 Gm. of fat, or 170 calories.

	household measurement	weight of portion
Milk, whole	1 cup	240 Gm.
Milk, evaporated	1/2 cup	120 Gm.
*Milk, powdered	1/4 cup	35 Gm.
*Buttermilk	1 cup	240 Gm.

*Add 2 fat exchanges if milk is fat-free.

TABLE 7–14. 2500 Calorie Diet.

2500 calories
(approximately)

carbohydrate	250 Gm.
protein	100 Gm.
fat	120 Gm.

Daily menu guide

The foods allowed in your diet should be selected from the seven exchange lists on this page. Menus should be planned on the basis of the menu guide given below. Foods in the same list are interchangeable, because, in the quantities specified, they provide approximately the same amounts of carbohydrate, protein, and fat. For example, when your menu calls for one bread exchange, any item in List 4 may be used in the amount stated. If two bread exchanges are allowed, double the specified amount or use a single exchange of *two* foods in List 4. Sample menus on the reverse side of this sheet illustrate correct use of the exchange lists.

BREAKFAST

2 fruit exchanges (List 3)
3 1/2 bread exchanges (List 4)
3 meat exchanges (List 5)
1 milk exchange (List 7)
3 fat exchanges (List 6)
Coffee or tea (any amount)

LUNCH

2 meat exchanges (List 5)
4 bread exchanges (List 4)
Vegetable(s) as desired (List 1)
1 fruit exchange (List 3)
1 milk exchange (List 7)
4 fat exchanges (List 6)
Coffee or tea (any amount)

DINNER

2 meat exchanges (List 5)
3 bread exchanges (List 4)
Vegetable(s) as desired (List 1)
1 vegetable exchange (List 2)
2 fruit exchanges (List 3)
1 milk exchange (List 7)
4 fat exchanges (List 6)
Coffee or tea (any amount)

BEDTIME FEEDING

(Only when directed by physician)
1/2 milk exchange   ⎞ will add
   (1/2 cup milk)   ⎬ approximately
1/2 bread exchange   ⎨ 120 calories to
   (2 crackers)   ⎠ daily diet

List 1 allowed as desired
(need not be measured)

Seasonings: Cinnamon, celery salt, garlic, garlic salt, lemon, mustard, mint, nutmeg, parsley, pepper, saccharin and other sugarless sweeteners, spices, vanilla, and vinegar.

Other Foods: Coffee or tea (without sugar or cream), fat-free broth, bouillon, unflavored gelatin, rennet tablets, sour or dill pickles, cranberries (without sugar), rhubarb (without sugar).

Vegetables: Group A—insignificant carbohydrate or calories. You may eat as much as desired of raw vegetable. If cooked vegetable is eaten, limit amount to 1 cup.

Asparagus	Lettuce
Broccoli	Mushrooms
Brussels sprouts	Okra
Cabbage	Peppers, green
Cauliflower	or red
Celery	Radishes
Chicory	Sauerkraut
Cucumbers	String beans
Eggplant	Summer squash
Escarole	Tomatoes
Greens: beet, chard, collard,	Watercress
dandelion, kale, mustard,	
spinach, turnip	

List 2 vegetable exchanges

Each portion supplies approximately 7 Gm. of carbohydrate and 2 Gm. of protein, or 36 calories.

Vegetables: Group B—One serving equals 1/2 cup, or 100 Gm.

Beets	Pumpkin
Carrots	Rutabagas
Onions	Squash, winter
Peas, green	Turnips

By permission of E. Lilly and Company, Indianapolis. Indiana.

TABLE 7–14. (Continued)

List 3 fruit exchanges

(fresh, dried, or canned without sugar)

Each portion supplies approximately 10 Gm. of carbohydrate, or 40 calories.

	household measurement	weight of portion
Apple	1 small (2″ diam.)	80 Gm.
Applesauce	1/2 cup	100 Gm.
Apricots, fresh	2 med.	100 Gm.
Apricots, dried	4 halves	20 Gm.
Banana	1/2 small	50 Gm.
Berries	1 cup	150 Gm.
Blueberries	2/3 cup	100 Gm.
Cantaloupe	1/4 (6″ diam.)	200 Gm.
Cherries	10 large	75 Gm.
Dates	2	15 Gm.
Figs, fresh	2 large	50 Gm.
Figs, dried	1 small	15 Gm.
Grapefruit	1/2 small	125 Gm.
Grapefruit juice	1/2 cup	100 Gm.
Grapes	12	75 Gm.
Grape juice	1/4 cup	60 Gm.
Honeydew melon	1/8 (7″)	150 Gm.
Mango	1/2 small	70 Gm.
Orange	1 small	100 Gm.
Orange juice	1/2 cup	100 Gm.
Papaya	1/3 med.	100 Gm.
Peach	1 med.	100 Gm.
Pear	1 small	100 Gm.
Pineapple	1/2 cup	80 Gm.
Pineapple juice	1/3 cup	80 Gm.
Plums	2 med.	100 Gm.
Prunes, dried	2	25 Gm.
Raisins	2 tbsp.	15 Gm.
Tangerine	1 large	100 Gm.
Watermelon	1 cup	175 Gm.

List 4 bread exchanges

Each portion supplies approximately 15 Gm. of carbohydrate and 2 Gm. of protein, or 68 calories.

	household measurement	weight of portion
Bread	1 slice	25 Gm.
Biscuit, roll	1 (2″ diam.)	35 Gm.
Muffin	1 (2″ diam.)	35 Gm.
Cornbread	1 1/2″ cube	35 Gm.
Flour	2 1/2 tbsp.	20 Gm.
Cereal, cooked	1/2 cup	100 Gm.
Cereal, dry (flakes or puffed)	3/4 cup	20 Gm.
Rice or grits, cooked	1/2 cup	100 Gm.
Spaghetti, noodles, etc.	1/2 cup	100 Gm.
Crackers, graham	2	20 Gm.
Crackers, oyster	20 (1/2 cup)	20 Gm.
Crackers, saltine	5	20 Gm.
Crackers, soda	3	20 Gm.
Crackers, round	6-8	20 Gm.
Vegetables		
Beans (Lima, navy, etc.), dry, cooked	1/2 cup	90 Gm.
Peas (split peas, etc.), dry, cooked	1/2 cup	90 Gm.
Baked beans, no pork	1/4 cup	50 Gm.
Corn	1/3 cup	80 Gm.
Parsnips	2/3 cup	125 Gm.
Potato, white, baked or boiled	1 (2″ diam.)	100 Gm.
Potatoes, white, mashed	1/2 cup	100 Gm.
Potatoes, sweet, or yams	1/4 cup	50 Gm.
Sponge cake, plain	1 1/2″ cube	25 Gm.
Ice cream (Omit 2 fat exchanges)	1/2 cup	70 Gm.

List 5 meat exchanges

Each portion supplies approximately 7 Gm. of protein and 5 Gm. of fat, or 73 calories. (30 Gm. equal 1 oz.)

	household measurement	weight of portion
Meat and poultry (beef, lamb, pork, liver, chicken, etc.) (med. fat)	1 slice (3″ x 2″ x 1/8″)	30 Gm.
Cold cuts	1 slice (4 1/2″ sq., 1/8″ thick)	45 Gm.
Frankfurter	1 (8-9 per lb.)	50 Gm.
Codfish, mackerel, etc.	1 slice (2″ x 2″ x 1″)	30 Gm.
Salmon, tuna, crab	1/4 cup	30 Gm.
Oysters, shrimp, clams	5 small	45 Gm.
Sardines	3 med.	30 Gm.
Cheese, cheddar, American	1 slice (3 1/2″ x 1 1/2″ x 1/4″)	30 Gm.
Cheese, cottage	1/4 cup	45 Gm.
Egg	1	50 Gm.
Peanut butter	2 tbsp.	30 Gm.

Limit peanut butter to one exchange per day unless allowance is made for carbohydrate in the diet plan.

List 6 fat exchanges

Each portion supplies approximately 5 Gm. of fat, or 45 calories.

	household measurement	weight of portion
Butter or margarine	1 tsp.	5 Gm.
Bacon, crisp	1 slice	10 Gm.
Cream, light	2 tbsp.	30 Gm.
Cream, heavy	1 tbsp.	15 Gm.
Cream cheese	1 tbsp.	15 Gm.
French dressing	1 tbsp.	15 Gm.
Mayonnaise	1 tsp.	5 Gm.
Oil or cooking fat	1 tsp.	5 Gm.
Nuts	6 small	10 Gm.
Olives	5 small	50 Gm.
Avocado	1/8 (4″ diam.)	25 Gm.

List 7 milk exchanges

Each portion supplies approximately 12 Gm. of carbohydrate, 8 Gm. of protein, and 10 Gm. of fat, or 170 calories.

	household measurement	weight of portion
Milk, whole	1 cup	240 Gm.
Milk, evaporated	1/2 cup	120 Gm.
*Milk, powdered	1/4 cup	35 Gm.
*Buttermilk	1 cup	240 Gm.

*Add 2 fat exchanges if milk is fat-free.

TABLE 7–15. 3000 Calorie Diet.

3000 calories (approximately)	carbohydrate	300 Gm.
	protein	130 Gm.
	fat	140 Gm.

Daily menu guide

The foods allowed in your diet should be selected from the seven exchange lists on this page. Menus should be planned on the basis of the menu guide given below. Foods in the same list are interchangeable, because, in the quantities specified, they provide approximately the same amounts of carbohydrate, protein, and fat. For example, when your menu calls for one bread exchange, any item in List 4 may be used in the amount stated. If two bread exchanges are allowed, double the specified amount or use a single exchange of *two* foods in List 4. Sample menus on the reverse side of this sheet illustrate correct use of the exchange lists.

BREAKFAST
2 fruit exchanges (List 3)
2 bread exchanges (List 4)
2 meat exchanges (List 5)
1 milk exchange (List 7)
3 fat exchanges (List 6)
Coffee or tea (any amount)

LUNCH
3 meat exchanges (List 5)
4 bread exchanges (List 4)
Vegetable(s) as desired (List 1)
2 fruit exchanges (List 3)
1 milk exchange (List 7)
2 fat exchanges (List 6)
Coffee or tea (any amount)

MIDAFTERNOON FEEDING
1 meat exchange (List 5)
1 bread exchange (List 4)
1/2 milk exchange (List 7)
1 fat exchange (List 6)

DINNER
3 meat exchanges (List 5)
4 bread exchanges (List 4)
Vegetable(s) as desired (List 1)
1 vegetable exchange (List 2)
2 fruit exchanges (List 3)
1 milk exchange (List 7)
3 fat exchanges (List 6)
Coffee or tea (any amount)

BEDTIME FEEDING
2 bread exchanges (List 4)
2 meat exchanges (List 5)
1 fat exchange (List 6)

List 1 allowed as desired
(need not be measured)

Seasonings: Cinnamon, celery salt, garlic, garlic salt, lemon, mustard, mint, nutmeg, parsley, pepper, saccharin and other sugarless sweeteners, spices, vanilla, and vinegar.

Other Foods: Coffee or tea (without sugar or cream), fat-free broth, bouillon, unflavored gelatin, rennet tablets, sour or dill pickles, cranberries (without sugar), rhubarb (without sugar).

Vegetables: Group A—insignificant carbohydrate or calories. You may eat as much as desired of raw vegetable. If cooked vegetable is eaten, limit amount to 1 cup.

Asparagus	Lettuce
Broccoli	Mushrooms
Brussels sprouts	Okra
Cabbage	Peppers, green
Cauliflower	or red
Celery	Radishes
Chicory	Sauerkraut
Cucumbers	String beans
Eggplant	Summer squash
Escarole	Tomatoes
Greens: beet, chard, collard,	Watercress
dandelion, kale, mustard,	
spinach, turnip	

List 2 vegetable exchanges

Each portion supplies approximately 7 Gm. of carbohydrate and 2 Gm. of protein, or 36 calories.

Vegetables: Group B—One serving equals 1/2 cup, or 100 Gm.

Beets	Pumpkin
Carrots	Rutabagas
Onions	Squash, winter
Peas, green	Turnips

By permission of E. Lilly and Company, Indianapolis. Indiana.

TABLE 7–15. (Continued)

List **3** fruit exchanges

(fresh, dried, or canned without sugar)

Each portion supplies approximately 10 Gm. of carbohydrate, or 40 calories.

	household measurement	weight of portion
Apple	1 small (2″ diam.)	80 Gm.
Applesauce	1/2 cup	100 Gm.
Apricots, fresh	2 med.	100 Gm.
Apricots, dried	4 halves	20 Gm.
Banana	1/2 small	50 Gm.
Berries	1 cup	150 Gm.
Blueberries	2/3 cup	100 Gm.
Cantaloupe	1/4 (6″ diam.)	200 Gm.
Cherries	10 large	75 Gm.
Dates	2	15 Gm.
Figs, fresh	2 large	50 Gm.
Figs, dried	1 small	15 Gm.
Grapefruit	1/2 small	125 Gm.
Grapefruit juice	1/2 cup	100 Gm.
Grapes	12	75 Gm.
Grape juice	1/4 cup	60 Gm.
Honeydew melon	1/8 (7″)	150 Gm.
Mango	1/2 small	70 Gm.
Orange	1 small	100 Gm.
Orange juice	1/2 cup	100 Gm.
Papaya	1/3 med.	100 Gm.
Peach	1 med.	100 Gm.
Pear	1 small	100 Gm.
Pineapple	1/2 cup	80 Gm.
Pineapple juice	1/3 cup	80 Gm.
Plums	2 med.	100 Gm.
Prunes, dried	2	25 Gm.
Raisins	2 tbsp.	15 Gm.
Tangerine	1 large	100 Gm.
Watermelon	1 cup	175 Gm.

List **4** bread exchanges

Each portion supplies approximately 15 Gm. of carbohydrate and 2 Gm. of protein, or 68 calories.

	household measurement	weight of portion
Bread	1 slice	25 Gm.
Biscuit, roll	1 (2″ diam.)	35 Gm.
Muffin	1 (2″ diam.)	35 Gm.
Cornbread	1 1/2″ cube	35 Gm.
Flour	2 1/2 tbsp.	20 Gm.
Cereal, cooked	1/2 cup	100 Gm.
Cereal, dry (flakes or puffed)	3/4 cup	20 Gm.
Rice or grits, cooked	1/2 cup	100 Gm.
Spaghetti, noodles, etc.	1/2 cup	100 Gm.
Crackers, graham	2	20 Gm.
Crackers, oyster	20 (1/2 cup)	20 Gm.
Crackers, saltine	5	20 Gm.
Crackers, soda	3	20 Gm.
Crackers, round	6-8	20 Gm.
Vegetables		
Beans (Lima, navy, etc.), dry, cooked	1/2 cup	90 Gm.
Peas (split peas, etc.), dry, cooked	1/2 cup	90 Gm.
Baked beans, no pork	1/4 cup	50 Gm.
Corn	1/3 cup	80 Gm.
Parsnips	2/3 cup	125 Gm.
Potato, white, baked or boiled	1 (2″ diam.)	100 Gm.
Potatoes, white, mashed	1/2 cup	100 Gm.
Potatoes, sweet, or yams	1/4 cup	50 Gm.
Sponge cake, plain	1 1/2″ cube	25 Gm.
Ice cream (Omit 2 fat exchanges)	1/2 cup	70 Gm.

List **5** meat exchanges

Each portion supplies approximately 7 Gm. of protein and 5 Gm. of fat, or 73 calories. (30 Gm. equal 1 oz.)

	household measurement	weight of portion
Meat and poultry (beef, lamb, pork, liver, chicken, etc.) (med. fat)	1 slice (3″ x 2″ x 1/8″)	30 Gm.
Cold cuts	1 slice (4 1/2″ sq., 1/8″ thick)	45 Gm.
Frankfurter	1 (8-9 per lb.)	50 Gm.
Codfish, mackerel, etc.	1 slice (2″ x 2″ x 1″)	30 Gm.
Salmon, tuna, crab	1/4 cup	30 Gm.
Oysters, shrimp, clams	5 small	45 Gm.
Sardines	3 med.	30 Gm.
Cheese, cheddar, American	1 slice (3 1/2″ x 1 1/2″ x 1/4″)	30 Gm.
Cheese, cottage	1/4 cup	45 Gm.
Egg	1	50 Gm.
Peanut butter	2 tbsp.	30 Gm.

Limit peanut butter to one exchange per day unless allowance is made for carbohydrate in the diet plan.

List **6** fat exchanges

Each portion supplies approximately 5 Gm. of fat, or 45 calories.

	household measurement	weight of portion
Butter or margarine	1 tsp.	5 Gm.
Bacon, crisp	1 slice	10 Gm.
Cream, light	2 tbsp.	30 Gm.
Cream, heavy	1 tbsp.	15 Gm.
Cream cheese	1 tbsp.	15 Gm.
French dressing	1 tbsp.	15 Gm.
Mayonnaise	1 tsp.	5 Gm.
Oil or cooking fat	1 tsp.	5 Gm.
Nuts	6 small	10 Gm.
Olives	5 small	50 Gm.
Avocado	1/8 (4″ diam.)	25 Gm.

List **7** milk exchanges

Each portion supplies approximately 12 Gm. of carbohydrate, 8 Gm. of protein, and 10 Gm. of fat, or 170 calories.

	household measurement	weight of portion
Milk, whole	1 cup	240 Gm.
Milk, evaporated	1/2 cup	120 Gm.
*Milk, powdered	1/4 cup	35 Gm.
*Buttermilk	1 cup	240 Gm.

*Add 2 fat exchanges if milk is fat-free.

166

statement 30

The utilization of oxygen during exercise is a function of the type of exercise and the state of training of the individual.

Introduction Astrand and Rhyming describe a test administered on a bicycle ergometer which is one method for the evaluation of endurance fitness outside the laboratory setting.[1] The test consists of measuring the heart rate during exercise. This particular exercise protocol calls for a submaximal exercise workload that elicits a continuous, steady heart rate.

The information gathered from this activity may be applied to several of the other statements. The score (milliliters of oxygen used per kilogram of body weight) can be used as a comparative figure for endurance fitness improvement and programming.

Procedure 1. Administer the test with the Monark ergometer as it is described by Astrand and Rhyming in the booklet provided with the purchase of the ergometer.

2. The chart below should be completed:

Age _____   Weight _____

Date			Heart Rate				Average
	1	2	3	4	5	6	
————	—	—	—	—	—	—	————
————	—	—	—	—	—	—	————

[1] P. O. Astrand and I. Rhyming, "A Nomogram for Calculation of Aerobic Capacity from Pulse Rate during Sub-Maximal Work," *Journal of Applied Physiology*, 7 (1954), 218–21.

167

TEST SUMMARY

Date _____ _____

Maximal Oxygen Consumption _____ _____

Corrected (VO$_2$ × age factor) _____ _____

Oxygen Consumption
(ml/kg/min) _____ _____

Fitness Category[2]
(see Statement 33) _____ _____

**Teaching
Methods**

Performance Objective

The student should be able to obtain a predicted oxygen consumption normalized for body weight as determined by the Astrand-Rhyming protocol and tables.

Teaching Hints
1. The instructor should take some time to train several interested students in the administration of this test. These students can give the test at any time during the school day and throughout the school year. The number of trained students will increase as more people are tested and become interested in the test.
2. The systolic blood pressure should be obtained during the fifth and sixth minutes of the exercise test.
3. If a bicycle ergometer is unavailable, a submaximal step test can be substituted (for example see Figure 7–2).

Discussion
1. Is this a difficult test compared to the 12-minute run or the Harvard Step Test? Are there some advantages to a submaximal test such as this?
2. How does the information from this test compare to the 12-minute run and the step test? How might the differences be explained?
3. List four methods for improving your ability to utilize oxygen.
4. Within what energy-source time period would you develop your program?

[2]Kenneth H. Cooper, *The New Aerobics* (New York: Bantam Books, 1970).

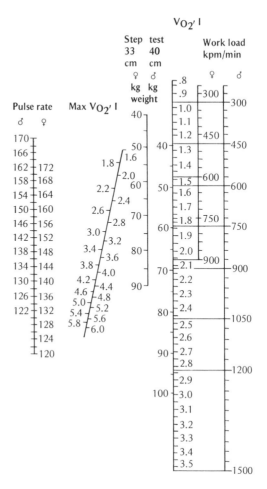

Figure 7–2. A nomogram for predicting oxygen uptake from heart rate data on step test or bicycle ergometer. From I. Astrand, "Aerobic Work Capacity in Men and Women with Special Reference to Age," *Acta Physiologica Scand.* 49 (Suppl 169), 1960. For the step test the following directions should be followed:

1. The stepping rate to a 15 inch step should be 22.5 per minute.
2. Obtain a steady state heart rate during the last minute of a six minute test, or immediately upon cessation of the test.
3. Draw a line between the heart rate value and the body weight figure (1 kg = 2.2 lbs). Read the estimated Max Vo₂ at the point of intersection of the line and the Max Vo₂ chart.

Materials 1. Monark bicycle ergometer. Quinton Instruments, 3051 44th Ave. West, Seattle, Wash. 98199.

2. Interval timer.

3. Stopwatch.

4. Metronome.

statement 31

When the exercise demand is greater than the aerobic capacity, the exercise will be short-term.

Introduction An activity so demanding that it is impossible to continue for more than two minutes is considered relative short-term exercise. The energy demands on the muscle in this type of activity are of such a magnitude that the muscle must use nonoxidative energy sources (see Statement 2). Upon depletion of these nonoxidative sources, the muscles are forced to stop contracting (the point of fatigue or exhaustion).

The aerobic capacity represents that maximum activity level that can be performed for at least five minutes. It is determined by the ability to supply oxygen to the working muscles and the ability of the muscles to utilize that oxygen for the energy production that is necessary for the activity. If the activity requires more energy than can be supplied by this oxidative system, the activity cannot be performed for a sustained period of time.

Energy supply is not the only cause of fatigue or exhaustion; other statements explore alternative reasons.

Procedure 1. Record the student's resting pulse and respiratory rates.
2. Pedal on the bicycle ergometer at 100 pedal revolutions per minute with a workload that produces a higher heart rate than the heart rate determined in Statement 30, the aerobic capacity level.
3. Record the exercise time.
4. Take a 10-second heart rate count immediately after stopping the exercise and multiply by six to give a good estimation of the heart rate during exercise.
5. Count the respiratory rate for one minute from the moment the student discontinues exercise. Recovery heart rates should be taken at one-minute intervals for three minutes.
6. Repeat this procedure at a higher work rate which will produce a quicker fatigue time. Record the exercise-time heart rates and respiratory rates as in (4) and (5) above.

Teaching Methods

Performance Objective

The student should be able to record the increases in heart and respiratory rate and observe or personally feel the maximal physical effort.

Teaching Hints
1. If a bicycle ergometer is unavailable, a nonoxidative response to exercise may be elicited by a fast step test, running up and down stairs, or sprinting on a playing field or in the gymnasium.
2. Plot the nonoxidative response in this statement using question 3 under Discussion.

Discussion
1. Why can nonoxidative-type activities be continued for only a short period of time?
2. Circle the nonoxidative type of activity: basketball, tennis, sprinting, swimming for ½ mile, weightlifting, jogging.
3. Diagram a nonoxidative response to exercise.

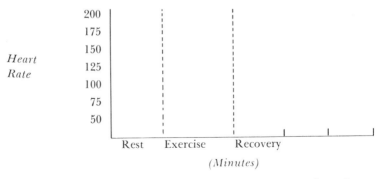

4. Why did the more strenuous workload induce fatigue faster than the less strenuous task, even though both work rates eventually caused you to stop the activity?

Materials
1. Bicycle ergometer.
2. Stethoscope and stopwatch (heart rate can be taken by feeling the carotid artery).

statement 32

Long-term exercise depends upon a constant supply of oxygen.

Introduction   While resting, very little oxygen is needed; consequently, the heart rate remains low. Upon the initiation of even moderate exercise, a very rapid increase in the heart rate is observed. This increase is necessary to supply the working muscles with enough oxygen for the appropriate production of energy.

As can be observed, the cardiovascular system serves to support the energy system by delivering enough oxygen for moderate exercise. This type of exercise, with oxygen, is referred to as oxidative (or aerobic).

Procedure   1. Plot the heart rate information gathered from the bicycle ergometer test at rest and during exercise on the diagram on p. 173 (Statement 30).
2. Superimpose upon this diagram the response of the nonoxidative exercise bout from Statement 31.

Teaching Methods   *Performance Objective*
The students should be able to plot a heart response to continuous and short-term exercise.

Teaching Hint
After plotting the heart rate responses, as obtained from the test on the bicycle, the discussion phase is the most important part of this statement. The concept that a leveling-off or steady state is important for any long-term activity must be discussed.

Discussion   1. With six months of training, what would you expect your heart rate response to be to the same workload?
2. Discuss heart rate response, oxygen uptake ability, and oxygen debt in terms of long-term physical activity.
3. What source of energy is utilized in long-term steady-state activity?
4. List four recreational sports that would promote improvement in the oxidative system.

172

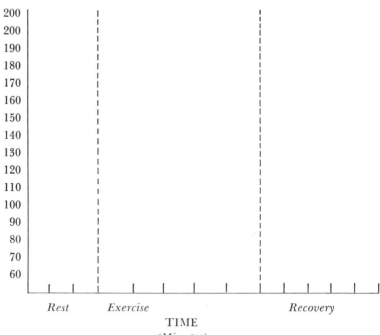

statement 33

An individual's aerobic capacity can be estimated by a 12-minute or a 1.5-mile running test.

Introduction

Oxygen consumption expressed in milliliters of oxygen per kilogram of body weight is perhaps the best test of endurance fitness available today. Kenneth Cooper, M.D., has developed a field test, based on scientific research, that can reasonably predict the ability of the body to utilize oxygen.[1] This type of data has also been developed for women.[2] The running test is based on laboratory treadmill data obtained from groups of varying fitness levels. The data show a linear relationship between the time of the run and the amount of oxygen consumed.

Aerobic capacity is a term that represents the maximum amount of oxygen that can be used by the body over a sustained activity period. This amount of oxygen reflects the functional state of fitness for prolonged activity. That is, in general, the higher the aerobic capacity, the more "in shape" a person is considered to be.

Procedure

1. Describe some precautions prior to administering this test such as the proper warm-up, running mechanics, breathing, intensity of the run, and recovery strategy.
2. Establish a measured course. This can be on a track, road, or in a gymnasium. Develop a conversion chart for laps into distance.
3. Record the time to run 1.5 miles or record the distance run in 12 minutes.
4. Refer to Tables 7–16 through 7–18 to determine the proper fitness category.
5. The predicted range of oxygen consumption can be found on Table 7–19.

Teaching Methods

Performance Objective

The student should be able to determine the endurance fitness level based on Cooper's indirect test.

[1]Kenneth H. Cooper, *The New Aerobics* (New York: Bantam Books, 1970).
[2]Mildred Cooper and Kenneth Cooper. *Aerobics for Women* (New York: Bantam Books, 1973).

TABLE 7–16. 1.5 Mile Test for Men.

FITNESS CATEGORY	AGE			
	Under 30	*30–39*	*40–49*	*50+*
I. Very Poor	16:30+	17:30+	18:30+	19:00+
II. Poor	16:30—	17:30—	18:30—	19:00—
	14:31	15:31	16:31	17:01
III. Fair	14:30—	15:30—	16:30—	17:00—
	12:01	13:01	14:01	14:31
IV. Good	12:00—	13:00—	14:00—	14:30—
	10:16	11:01	11:39	12:01
V. Excellent*	<10:15	<11:00	<11:38	<12:00

†No separate chart is provided for women because available data are still too tentative.

*For military personnel, the Excellent requirements are 15–30 seconds faster.

< Means less than.

From Kenneth H. Cooper, *The New Aerobics*. New York: Bantam Books, 1970.

TABLE 7–17. 12-Minute Test for Men (Distance in miles covered in 12 minutes).

FITNESS CATEGORY	AGE			
	Under 30	*30–39*	*40–49*	*50+*
I. Very Poor	<1.0	<.95	<.85	<.80
II. Poor	1.0 –1.24	.95–1.14	.85–1.04	.80– .99
III. Fair	1.25–1.49	1.15–1.39	1.05–1.29	1.0 –1.24
IV. Good	1.50–1.74	1.40–1.64	1.30–1.54	1.25–1.49
V. Excellent	1.75+	1.65+	1.55+	1.50+

< Means less than.

From Kenneth H. Cooper, *The New Aerobics*. New York: Bantam Books, 1970.

TABLE 7–18. 12 Minute Test for Women (Distance in miles covered in 12 minutes).

FITNESS CATEGORY	AGE			
	Under 30	*30–39*	*40–49*	*50+*
I. Very Poor	<.95	<.85	<.75	<.65
II. Poor	.95–1.14	.85–1.04	.75–.94	.65–.84
III. Fair	1.15–1.34	1.05–1.24	.95–1.14	.85–1.04
IV. Good	1.35–1.64	1.25–1.54	1.15–1.44	1.05–1.34
V. Excellent	1.65+	1.55+	1.45+	1.35+

*Preliminary chart based on limited data.

< Means less than.

From Mildred Cooper and Kenneth H. Cooper, *Aerobics for Women*. New York: Bantam Books, 1973.

TABLE 7–19.   **Fitness Categories Based upon Oxygen Consumption (ml/kg/min).**

FITNESS CATEGORY	OXYGEN CONSUMPTION (ml/kg/min)			
	Under 30	*30–39*	*40–49*	*50+*
I. Very Poor	<25.0	<25.0	<25.0	
II. Poor	25.0–33.7	25.0–30.1	25.0–26.4	<25.0
III. Fair	33.8–42.5	30.2–39.1	26.5–35.4	25.0–33.7
IV. Good	42.6–51.5	39.2–48.0	35.5–45.0	33.8–43.0
V. Excellent	51.6+	48.1+	45.1+	43.1+

< Means less than.
From Kenneth H. Cooper. *The New Aerobics.* New York: Bantam Books, 1970.

Teaching Hints

1. It must be pointed out that the time for the run or the distance covered is the primary determinant of aerobic capacity. If the student gets tired and wishes to stop this may be done, but a walking pace would be maintained. Initially, most students will do poorly on these tests because of faulty running mechanics and a lack of knowledge of pace.

2. This test forms the basis of two other statements; consequently, it must be administered early in the school year. Also, it can form the basis of understanding the relationship between "fitness levels," body fat, resting heart rate, somatotype, etc.

Discussion   1. Try to get the students to discuss the "limiting factor" to their performance.

2. Complete the fitness categories for the following subjects:

Subject	*Sex*	*Age*	*Distance*	*Fitness Category*
A	M	34	1.30 mi	_____
B	M	52	1.55 mi	_____
C	F	19	1.10 mi	_____
D	F	46	1.20 mi	_____
E	M	19	0.95 mi	_____

Materials   A measured running course and Tables 7–16 through 7–19.

statement 34

Heart rate during an activity indicates the level of energy expenditure.

Introduction Exercise physiologists have found that with progressively increasing workloads there exists a near linear relationship between heart rate and oxygen consumption. This is true, however, only between 50 to 90 percent of the maximal heart rate. As a result, the pulse rate can be used as a practical method to find energy expenditure levels of endurance fitness.

The purpose of this lesson is to allow the student to determine the energy requirement of some daily activities simply by determining the heart rate for that activity.

Procedure 1. Take the heart rate while participating in four or five different physical activities.
2. Locate the oxygen uptake in liters per minute on the graph (Figure 7–3) presented by drawing a line from the HR to the slope line, then dropping a line to the horizontal axis.
3. Multiply the V_{O_2} by 5 calories (5 calories is the energy gained by the burning of one liter of oxygen).
4. Multiply this figure by the total time of the activity to get the total caloric expenditure.
5. Complete the following chart:

Activity	Heart Rate	Oxygen Uptake	Caloric Factor	Calories per Minute	Total Time of Activity	Total Caloric Expenditure
1. Riding Ergometer	133	2.2	5	11	5	55
2.			5			
3.			5			
4.			5			
5.			5			

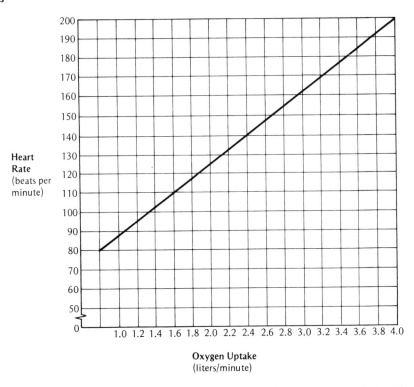

Figure 7–3. The relationship between heart rate and oxygen uptake. *Note:* The relationship between heart rate and oxygen uptake is dependent upon age, sex, work rate, and training level. Obviously, this figure should only be used as an approximation to the true relationships.

6. Using the formula 220 — age (use 226 for females), determine the heart rate range between 50 percent and 90 percent of maximum. For example, for a 16-year-old male student:

$$(220 - 16) \times .5 = 102$$

$$(220 - 16) \times .9 = 183$$

For this student Figure 7–3 would be accurate between HR of 102 to 183.

Teaching Methods

Performance Objective

The student should be able to calculate the energy requirement of several different physical activities by determining the heart rate during each activity.

Teaching Hints:

1. Make some suggestions for activities such as riding the ergometer, walking slowly, walking fast, jogging, sprinting, running upstairs,

lifting weights, etc., and then allow the students some time to complete the various activities.

2. Make the point that the resting heart rate is not an accurate estimation of energy cost because it does not fall between 50 and 90 percent of maximum HR.

3. It has been suggested that a workout should be intense enough to utilize at least 400 calories. Using the information calculated in Procedure 5, what time commitment is necessary for each activity to use at least 400 calories?

$$\text{Time to use 400 Calories} = \frac{400 \text{ Calories}}{\text{Cal/Min}}$$

For example:

$$\text{Riding a bicycle ergometer} = \frac{400 \text{ Calories}}{11 \text{ Cal/Min}} = 36.4 \text{ min}$$

Discussion
1. Is there a relationship between workload, heart rate, and energy cost for your own tests?
2. How do you suppose Cooper[1] established the aerobic point system?
3. How long could a person work at HR of 180, 140, 120, or 100?

Materials
1. Figure 7–3.

---

[1]Kenneth Cooper, *The New Aerobics* (New York: Bantam Books, 1970).

statement 35

The nonoxidative energy production capacity can be measured and related to several health and fitness and motor performance criteria.

Introduction According to Statement 3, the exercise time periods I–III are considered primarily nonoxidative (for exercises lasting up to 2 minutes). During these periods, high levels of intense activity can be performed with a high production of lactic acid (a barometer of nonoxidative energy production).

To assess this energy component, a simple test of stair running has been suggested by Margaria and Rovelli.[1] The power productions, in foot-pounds per second, can be related to somatotype, aerobic capacity, grip strength, sports activities, or whatever the imagination suggests.

Procedure 1. The subject should stand 6 feet from a flight of stairs. When ready, the steps should be ascended two at a time as quickly as possible.

2. The stopwatch will be started when the runner touches the fourth step and stopped when the twelfth step is reached. Three trials may be taken. The best time will be recorded.

   a. Best time of the three trials_____.

   b. Height of the steps in inches _____.

   c. Weight of the individual _____.

3. The formula for the determination of "nonoxidative" power:

$$\text{Nonoxidative Power} = \frac{W \times D}{t}$$

Where:

W = Weight of the person

D = Vertical height (in feet) between the fourth and twelfth step

t = Best time from the fourth to the twelfth step

[1] R. Margaria, P. Aghemo, and E. Rovelli, "Measurement of Muscular Power (Anaerobic) in Man," *Journal of Applied Physiology*, 21 (1966), 1664.

4. As an example, the test is scored as follows:

$$W = 155 \text{ lbs}$$

$$D = 8 \text{ steps} \times 8.5 \text{ in} = 5.66 \text{ ft}$$

$$t = 1.6 \text{ sec}$$

Nonoxidative power $= 155 \times 6.66 = 876$ foot pounds/seconds.

Teaching Methods

Performance Objective

The student should be able to measure nonoxidative power by Margaria's method.

Teaching Hints

1. Mark off the steps with some type of indicator so that the students take them two at a time. This will also be of value to the timer.
2. Demonstrate the use of the formula.
3. A most important consideration is to relate this information to sports participation, somatotype, aerobic capacity, etc. Graph the relationship between aerobic capacity and nonoxidative capacity.
4. There are some dangerous elements related to the performance of this statement so extra care should be exhibited.

Discussion

1. What type of training program will develop the nonoxidative capacity?
2. Discuss the relationships studied (i.e., power activities to somatotype; power to percent body fat, power to speed).
3. What implications does a high or low nonoxidative power score have for an individual?
4. What types of power activities demand nonoxidative energy sources?

Materials

Stairs and stopwatch.

chapter 8

Energy Support Systems

statement 36

Maximal external respiration is a measure of the capacity
of the lungs to inhale and exhale air.

Introduction

Before more accurate techniques were available, vital capacity, the volume of gas that can be exhaled by a maximal voluntary effort following full inspiration, was considered as a predictor of endurance performance capability. Actually, the lungs function only as a bellows based on some very simple mechanical principles, and serve as a dynamic reservoir for air flow. This external phase of physiology, regarding the lungs, is secondary to the internal phase which occurs at the tissue level.

Vital capacity, especially if impaired, is important to physical fitness; however, little difference in performance should be expected if the vital capacity measures are within normal ranges. Usually a decrease in vital capacity indicates a reduction in functioning lung tissue, as occurs in patients with pneumonia, carcinoma, fibrosis, pulmonary congestion, or respiratory muscular weakness. Physical training programs usually result in only minimal increased vital capacity.

Procedure

1. Administer a test to measure vital capacity (VC).
2. Using the nomograms provided in Figures 8–1 and 8–2 (see pages 186–87) predict vital capacity.
3. According to Comroe et al., a vital capacity 20 percent below predicted is considered abnormal.[1]
4. Discuss the relationship between the previous three steps.
5. To determine the relationship of VC to endurance fitness, plot VC and the estimated VO_2 from the bicycle ergometer test (Statement 30) for all students in the class.

Teaching Methods

Performance Objective

The student should be able to determine vital capacity.

---

[1]J. H. Comroe, R. E. Forster, A. B. Dubois, W. A. Briscee, and E. Carlson, *The Lung* (Chicago: The Year Book Publishers, Inc., 1960).

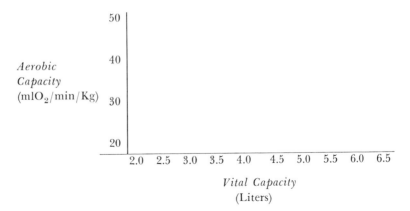

1. If a spirometer, vitalometer, vitalor, or respirometer is unavailable, a simple apparatus can be made with a large jar, tubing, and stopper from the science department. The student should blow into the jar and the amount of water displaced should be measured.
2. The following is an illustration of the formula for the prediction of normal vital capacity ranges. Student A has a measured vital capacity of 3.2 liters. The nomogram predicts a vital capacity of 3.8 liters.

$$\text{VC at } 20\% \text{ of Predicted} = 3.8 \times .8$$
$$= 3.2 \text{ L}$$

Consequently, Student A's vital capacity is at the lowest point of the normal range.
3. A selected student might gather these data for the total class.

Discussion

1. Is the student's VC within the normal range? If not, can it be accounted for?
2. Is VC related to endurance fitness (VO_2)? If not, how do you account for this? What are the other bodily systems which influence fitness levels?
3. How does the pulmonary system adapt to training?
4. What are the effects of altitude, smoking, and air pollution on respiration?

Materials

1. A small pocket-size dry spirometer can be purchased from J. A. Preston, 71 Fifth Ave., New York, N.Y. 10003, for $108.40.
2. A vitalometer or respirometer can be purchased from Warren E. Collins, Inc., 20 Weed Rd., Braintree, Mass. 02184.

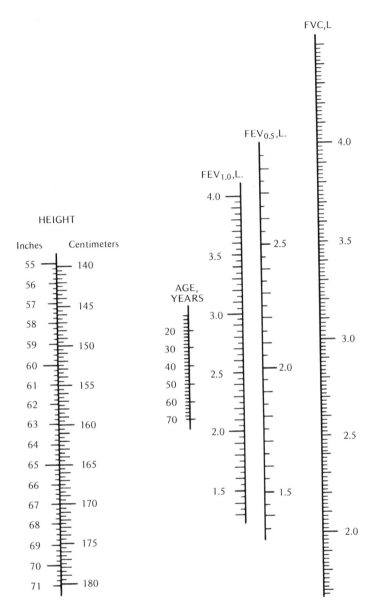

Figure 8–1. Prediction of vital capacity in normal females. From Kory, Smith, and Callahan.

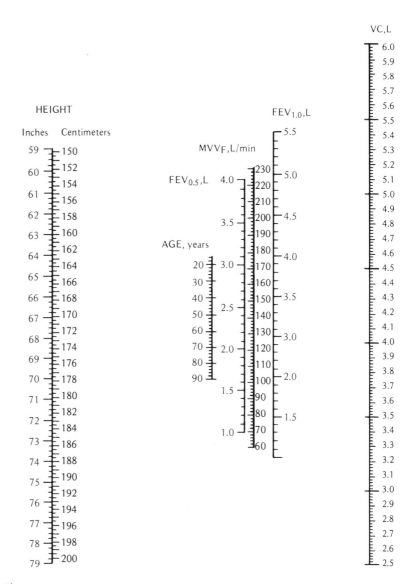

Figure 8–2. Prediction of vital capacity in normal males. From R.F. Kory, R. Callahan, H. G. Boren, and J.C. Snyder, The Veterans Administration-Army Cooperative Study of Pulmonary Function: I. Clinical Spirometry in Normal Men. *American Journal of Medicine*, 30 (1961), 243–58.

statement 37

Alteration in the response of the cardiovascular system at rest, during exercise, and in recovery is likely to be a function of the level of endurance fitness.

Introduction   Certain beneficial changes occur in the body as a result of regular physical activity. Exercise physiologists call these alterations *training effects*. Heart rate changes at rest, during exercise, and in recovery are reported in the scientific literature as a result of training.

A lower resting heart rate is a known adaptation to a regular physical training program, as is a lower exercising heart rate during a standard workload. During recovery from exercise, it is known that the trained individual has a faster return to resting conditions.

The Harvard Step Test[1] can be administered as described in the Procedure. This test was developed at the Harvard Fatigue Laboratory in 1943 as a measure of cardiovascular-respiratory efficiency. It uses recovery heart rate as an indicator of fitness. If the data gathered from this test is plotted on the graph on page 190, the students should be able to understand the variation in heart rate for the different fitness levels at rest, during exercise, and in recovery.

Procedure   1. For the Harvard Step Test the subject steps up and down thirty times a minute on a bench 18 inches high (the usual height of a gymnasium bench). Each time, the subject should step all the way up on the bench with the body erect. Stepping is done in four counts.

2. The exercise continues for exactly 5 minutes unless the subject is forced to stop sooner owing to exhaustion. In either case, the duration of the exercise in seconds is recorded: the maximum number of seconds is 300 for the full 5-minute period.

3. Immediately after completing the exercise the student must take a 10-second pulse count and multiply by 6 for the minute rate. This will give a HR that is reasonably close to the rate while exercising.

[1]L. Breuha, C. W. Heath and A. Graybiel, "Step Test: Simple Method of Measuring Physical Fitness for Hard Muscular Work in Adult Men," *Review of Canadian Biology*, 2 (1943), 86.

Resting HR _____

Post-Exercise HR _____

4. Next, the student should sit and take a pulse rate from 1 to 1½, 2 to 2½, 3 to 3½, 4 to 4½, and 5 to 5½ minutes after stepping ceases.

RECOVERY HEART RATE CHART (× 2 for minute rate)

1st Min	*2nd Min*	*3rd Min*	*4th Min*	*5th Min*
_____	_____	_____	_____	_____

5. The physical efficiency index (PEI) is computed, utilizing the following formula:

$$PEI = \frac{\text{Duration of Exercise in sec} \times 100}{\text{Sum of the First Three Minute Pulse Counts}}$$

6. On the basis of about 8,000 college students tested, the following norms were prepared:

Below 55—Poor physical condition
  55–64—Low average
  65–79—High average
  80–89—Good
Above 90—Excellent

7. Plot the HR response of the three fitness categories on the graph on the top of page 190.

Teaching Methods

Performance Objective

The student should be able to determine the fitness level based on the established norms, and plot the class heart rate response at rest, during exercise, and in recovery.

Teaching Hints
1. Explain carefully the procedures of the test, particularly the taking of recovery HR.
2. Use a metronome and/or have a student beat the cadence on a metal chair with a metal object.
3. The instructor should encourage and motivate the students. Shout out the time worked and the time remaining.
4. After the exercise and the 5-minute recovery period, illustrate the use of the formula. The following is an example of a subject who

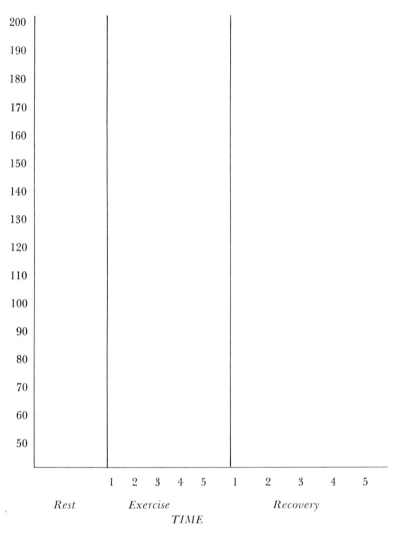

completed the entire period in 300 seconds when the recovery period pulse counts were 150, 100, and 70 for the first three minutes:

$$150$$
$$100$$
$$70$$
$$\overline{320}$$

$$\text{PEI} = \frac{300 \times 100}{320}$$

$$\text{PEI} = 94$$

$$\text{PEI} = \text{Excellent}$$

5. After the PEI has been determined select three students to record the HR information for the poor category, the average category, and the good and excellent category. Have the students make a chart

similar to the one below and then graph the results as in Procedure 7.

Category	HR (Rest)	HR (Exercise)	Recovery Minutes
			1 2 3 4 5
Poor			
Average			
Good			
Excellent			

6. An alternative step test is suggested for women by McArdle et al.[1] This is a 3-minute step test (22 steps per minute or at a cadence of 88 beats per minute). The heart rate is taken for 15 seconds immediately upon the completion of the exercise. See Table 8–1 for norms.

Discussion   1. How do you explain the lower heart rates for the higher fitness levels?
2. How does an individual alter the heart rate response to exercise?
3. Is oxygen uptake related to cardiovascular factors?

TABLE 8–1.   Percentile Norms for Recovery Heart Rate Following 3-Minute Step Test for Women. From W.D. McArdle, G.S. Pechar, F.I. Katch, and J.R. Magel, "Percentile Norms for a Valid Step Test in College Women," Research Quarterly, 44 (1973), 198–500.

PERCENTILE	5–20 SEC HEART RATE, BPM	PERCENTILE	5–20 SEC HEART RATE BPM
100	128	45	168
95	140	40	170
90	148	35	171
85	152	30	172
80	156	25	176
75	158	20	180
70	160	15	182
65	162	10	184
60	163	5	184
55	164	0	216
50	166		

(N = 300)

[1]W. D. McArdle, G. S. Pechar, F. I. Katch, and J. R. Magel, "Percentile Norms for a Valid Step Test in College Women," *Research Quarterly*, 44 (1973), 198–500.

4. What are the neural and hormonal control mechanisms of the heart during rest, exercise, and recovery?
5. How many daily heartbeats does a person with a resting HR of 60 have compared to a person with a resting heart rate of 80? Weekly? Yearly?

Materials
1. Metronome.
2. Some device to amplify the metronome sounds: a loudspeaker or a beating device.

statement **38**

To improve or maintain endurance fitness, specified weekly levels of exercise are needed.

Introduction Dr. Kenneth Cooper has assigned points to activities according to metabolic demand.[1] For example, a one-mile run completed in a time of between 14:30 and 20:00 minutes has been assigned a value of 1 point, while the same run accomplished in a time of 6:30 to 8:00 will gain the participant 5 points. Dr. Cooper has provided such equivalent points to a variety of "aerobic" activities including running, cycling, swimming, dancing, handball, basketball, tennis, etc. This point system is an extremely convenient method for determining the proper amount of activity for the development or maintenance of endurance fitness based on levels of previous training.

When the following illustrated chart of weekly activity is completed, the students should be able to determine the number of points earned. Those who are very active should continue their present efforts, while those who earned only a very few points should begin a progressive program to develop a higher endurance fitness level.

Procedure 1. The students should complete the chart below using the information from the appendix in either *The New Aerobics* or *Aerobics for Women*.[2]

Day	Activity	Time	Distance	Points
			Actual Points	
			GOAL	

[1] Kenneth H. Cooper, *The New Aerobics* (New York: Bantam Books, 1970).
[2] Mildred and Kenneth Cooper, *Aerobics for Women* (New York: Bantam Books, 1973).

2. To improve fitness, each student must establish a goal. This goal is developed from the present level of fitness based on the 12-minute test (Statement 33) and/or Astrand's Bicycle Ergometer test (see Statement 30). From our experience with aerobic programming, the following combination of points per fitness category seems appropriate for high school and college students (Table 8–2).

It should be pointed out that this program should only serve as a guide. Some students will reach the 24–30 point level earlier or later than suggested.

Teaching Methods

Performance Objective

The student should be able to determine the number of points of aerobic activity obtained per week based on the work of Cooper.

Teaching Hints

1. Copies of *The New Aerobics* and/or *Aerobics for Women* should be available in the instructor's office or library.
2. Procedure 1 can be completed in class or for homework. A place to start would be to determine the number of points obtained from the 12-minute or the 1.5-mile test.

TABLE 8–2.   Activity Points Necessary Per Week for Each Fitness Category

Week	Very poor & poor	Fair	Good & Excellent
1	5	12–15	30
2	7–10	12–15	
3	7–10	15–18	
4	10–12	18–20	
5	12–15	18–22	
6	12–15	20–25	
7	15–18	22–88	
8	18–20	24–30	
9	20–22		
10	20–24		
11	22–28		
12	24–30		
13			
14			
15			
16			

Adapted from Kenneth H. Cooper, *The New Aerobics.* New York: Bantam Books, 1970.

3. For a better understanding, have the students complete the following activities.

Activity	Distance	Time	Points
Running	1 mile	11:00	
Running	2.2 miles	17:00	
Running	3.7 miles	30:00	
Walking	1 mile	16:00	
Basketall		30:00	
Bike Riding	4 miles	20:00	
Swimming	800 yds	20:00	
Bowling		3 Strings	
Tennis		3 Sets	

Discussion
1. Why doesn't Cooper include bowling on his list of points?
2. Is the number of points you obtain per week in harmony with your fitness level? For example, if you get 50 points per week, is your fitness category excellent?

Materials   The appendixes from the Coopers' books.

statement 39

Aerobic fitness training programs can be based on four considerations.

Introduction

Wilmore and Haskell list the following four considerations for developing endurance fitness: (1) type of activity, (2) frequency of participation, (3) duration of each day's activity, and (4) the intensity of the performance.[1] The exact combination of these four factors to result in the most appropriate fitness program is difficult to prescribe. However, the above factors used in combination with the aerobic fitness concept of Cooper[2] provides a functional method to design individual endurance fitness programs.

Procedure

1. In light of the previously determined fitness category and the number of fitness points prescribed per week, fill in the following chart (use data from Statement 38).

Date	Activity	Distance	Time	Points

2. Describe your activity patterns in terms of the four considerations for developing an endurance fitness training program.

[1]Jack H. Wilmore and William J. Haskell, "Use of Heart Rate Energy Expenditure Relationship in the Individualized Prescription of Exercise," *American Journal Clinical Nutrition*, 24 (1971), 1186–92.
[2]Kenneth H. Cooper, *The New Aerobics* (New York: Bantam Books, 1970).

Principle	*Description*
Type of Activity (What activity?)	_____
Frequency (How often?)	_____
Duration (How long each time?)	_____
Intensity (What heart rate?)	_____

Teaching Methods

Performance Objectives

The students should be able to develop an aerobic fitness training program based on the appropriate fitness level and evaluate their personal fitness programs based upon the four stated considerations.

Teaching Hint

Students may have some difficulty understanding how to locate activities and appropriate points for the distance and/or time. Small groups of students helping each other is one effective method of class organization.

Discussion

1. List in order of preference four activities for promoting endurance fitness which you would include in your program.
2. If you could not participate in those activities listed above what alternatives would be available? Would these alternatives be as effective for promoting endurance fitness?
3. List the one reason why an aerobic fitness program would not work in your case.
4. List one method of overcoming the reason in the above statement.

statement 40

Cardiac response to exercise is directly proportional to the intensity of the workload and can be used to assess cardiovascular fitness.

Introduction

Graded exercise testing (GXT) has recently become popular as an assessment technique to identify persons with possible cardiovascular malfunctions. The GXT, when used in conjunction with electrocardiograph monitoring, can provide the physician, physical educator, and subject with some valuable data not readily detected in the resting state regarding the functional capacity of the heart.

Unfortunately, most schools do not have the personnel and equipment available to conduct GXT with electrocardiograph monitoring. The national YMCA has suggested a procedure involving increasingly progressive workloads for the assessment of cardiac response to exercise stress.[1] The test is described in Figure 8–3 and the methods for scoring in Figure 8–4. When administered over a period of time, the test allows the subject to assess the response of the cardiovascular system to exercise by observing the slope of the heart rates.

Procedure

1. Figure 8–3 and 8–4 provide the directions for the administration of this test.

Teaching Methods

Performance Objective

The student should be able to plot the response of the heart rate to three different exercise demands and to determine maximal oxygen consumption.

Teaching Hints

1. It is necessary to train some students to administer this test. The bicycle ergometer can be kept in a room other than the primary teaching station.
2. Figure 8–4 shows the scoring of the test demonstrated on one of the authors. The workload was set at 300 kilogrammeter (kgm) for the

[1]*The Y's Way to Physical Fitness*, C. R. Myers, L. A. Golding, and W. E. Sinning, eds. (Emmaus, Pa.: Rodale Press, 1973).

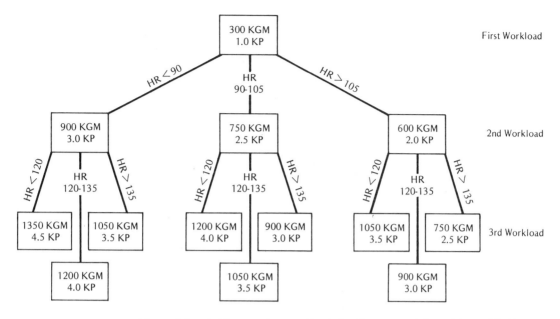

Figure 8–3. Guide to setting workloads for fitness test. Adapted from C.R. Myers, L.A. Golding, and W.E. Sinning (eds.), *The Y's Way to Physical Fitness.* Emmaus, Pa.: Rodale Press, 1973.

initial 3 minutes. Heart rate was taken at the end of the third minute and was less than 90 heart rate. The second workload was 900 kgm as determined by the flowchart from Figure 8–3. Because the initial HR was less than 90, the strategy dictated a flow to the lefthand column. The third setting was determined from the third minute of the second workload, which found the HR to be within the 120 to 135 range. Consequently, a 1200 kgm workload was selected.

3. The HR for the second and third workloads were plotted on Figure 8–4. Barring errors in the administration of the test, the subject improved in the response to the three demands from October to April.

4. To determine the $\dot{V}O_2$, follow the directions given in Figure 8–3. There, the subject's maximum heart rate was determined: 220 − 38 = 182. A horizontal line was drawn from the righthand heart rate column to the point where the exercise heart rate line meets. Drop a line from that point to the baseline. Maximum $\dot{V}O_2$ is given in liters per minute. To obtain the predicted $\dot{V}O_2$ in ml/kg, use the data from Statement 30. The subject illustrated predicts a $\dot{V}O_2$ value of 4.0 L. When applied to Table 8–3 a value of 56 ml/kg/min is given.

Figure 8-4. Scoring directions for fitness test. Adapted from C.R. Myers, L.A. Golding, and W.E. Sinning (eds.), *The Y's Way to Physical Fitness*. Emmaus, Pa.: Rodale Press, 1973.

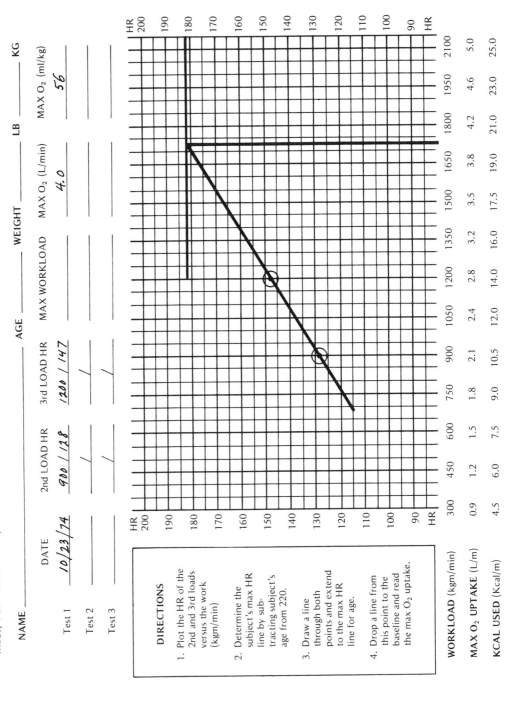

NAME _____

	DATE	2nd LOAD HR	3rd LOAD HR	AGE ___	WEIGHT ___	MAX O₂ (L/min)	LB ___	MAX O₂ (ml/kg)	KG ___
					MAX WORKLOAD	4.0		56	
Test 1	$10/23/74$	$900 / 128$	$1200 / 147$						
Test 2		/	/						
Test 3		/	/						

DIRECTIONS

1. Plot the HR of the 2nd and 3rd loads versus the work (kgm/min)

2. Determine the subject's max HR line by subtracting subject's age from 220.

3. Draw a line through both points and extend to the max HR line for age.

4. Drop a line from this point to the baseline and read the max O₂ uptake.

WORKLOAD (kgm/min)	300	450	600	750	900	1050	1200	1350	1500	1650	1800	1950	2100
MAX O₂ UPTAKE (L/m)	0.9	1.2	1.5	1.8	2.1	2.4	2.8	3.2	3.5	3.8	4.2	4.6	5.0
KCAL USED (Kcal/m)	4.5	6.0	7.5	9.0	10.5	12.0	14.0	16.0	17.5	19.0	21.0	23.0	25.0

Discussion   1. Are there any advantages to a graded exercise test such as the present GXT compared to the single-stage workload test used in Statement 30?
2. How do you explain the heart rate changes with increased demands?
3. If the slope of your test shifts to the right, how do you explain that?

Materials   1. The same equipment as used in Statement 30.
2. Charts are provided here.

statement 41

> There is a threshold intensity, above which there will be an improvement in endurance fitness.

Introduction   It has been established that unless exercise is strenuous enough, little or no endurance fitness will result. In general, exercise physiologists suggest that a work rate that elevates the heart rate to 70 percent of maximum (about 140 beats per minute) is necessary to induce training adaptations. Heart rate is a good indicator of exercise stress because it has been determined that heart rate corresponds to several metabolic barometers of exercise effort (e.g., oxygen uptake, cardiac output, respiratory rate, etc.).

It is well-known that the body has a reserve capacity for activity, thus it is possible to perform several low levels of activity even with no training. Only when the activity level is at a high enough intensity (threshold) does the body need to adapt its present capacity for exercise. The body adapts only in relation to the stress imposed during the exercise session. This statement should allow the student to experience the intensity of exercise necessary to induce a training adaptation.

Procedure   1. Three methods are presented to aid the student in determining the exercise heart rate threshold for the promotion of endurance fitness.
2. The Exercise Intensity Threshold (EIT) has been developed by deVries and defined by him as "the threshold below which no cardiovascular fitness improvement will result."[1]

$$EIT = \frac{\text{Oxygen Uptake (ml/kg)}}{100} \times (\text{Max HR} - \text{Rest HR}) + \text{Res HR}$$

3. Morehouse has suggested the following formulae:[2]

Men: (220 — Age) (% of Max HR Desired)

Women: (226 — Age) (% of Max HR Desired)

[1] Herbert deVries, "Exercise Intensity Threshold for the Improvement of Cardiovascular Function in Older Men," *Geriatrics*, 26 (1971), 94–101.
[2] Lawrence Morehouse, *Executive Fitness Clinics: A Multimedia Report* (Minneapolis: AAHPER, 1973).

4. Karvonen has established the following formula:[3]

$$HR = (Max\ HR - Rest\ HR)\ (.6) + Rest\ HR$$

Teaching Methods

Performance Objective

Determine the exercise heart rate that would be necessary for promoting a training effect utilizing the three different threshold methods.

Teaching Hints

1. This lesson could be integrated with a unit on cardiovascular disease and how to use exercise as a preventive technique.
2. The oxygen consumption for the deVries formula may be obtained from the 12-minute or 1.5-mile test or by the use of a bicycle ergometer.

Discussion

1. List the method and the threshold HR determined:

Method   *HR*

1.

2.

3.

2. What is the range of threshold heart rates calculated from the three tests?
3. What fitness levels do you think would require higher threshold levels? Why?
4. What activity might you suggest for the 65-year-old person based on his or her threshold intensity? A 19-year-old based on his or her threshold intensity?

[3]M. J. Karvonen, "Effect of Vigorus Exercise on the Heart," in *Work and the Heart*, F. Rosenbaum and E. Belknap, eds. (New York: P. B. Hoeber, Inc., 1959). See also J. A. Davis, "Accuracy of the Karvonen Method for Determination of Exercise Intensity," (Knoxville, Tennessee: American College Sports Medicine, 1974).

statement 42

The heart rate during exercise is an important barometer
of appropriate stress.

Introduction   Exercise physiologists have reported that appropriate stress must be applied to produce the desired training effects. In Statement 41, an exercise threshold was calculated based on the factors of age, resting heart rate, and/or fitness levels. One of the four considerations for an endurance training program in Statement 39 was intensity of activity. The monitoring of heart rate is an excellent barometer indicating intensity.

    This statement should allow the students to perform an endurance exercise while monitoring the heart rate. At the conclusion of the exercise period they should be able to plot the exercise intensity and determine whether or not the work was appropriate to their fitness level.

Procedure   1. The instructor must select a form of endurance work. One group might play basketball or volleyball, monitoring the HR every 1 to 2 minutes. Another might jog or walk. One method of group supervision is for the instructor to conduct an interval training session based on a work-rest ratio of 1:1. For this, the students will run in place for 30 seconds. Five seconds after they have completed the exercise session, the instructor will provide a 10-second period for heart rate monitoring. The remaining 15 seconds of the rest period will be for converting the 10-second heart rate into the minute rate (multiply by 6) and recording in the space provided.
2. The instructor should carefully explain how to take the pulse count at the neck for the 10-second period.
3. The student should list the appropriate threshold heart rate. (Statement 41).
4. Record the minute heart rates in the chart below.

204

Activity	1	2	3	4	5	5	6	7	8	9	10

1.

2.

3.

4.

5.

5. For any one activity plot the exercise heart rate on the graph below. Draw a line through the threshold heart rate.

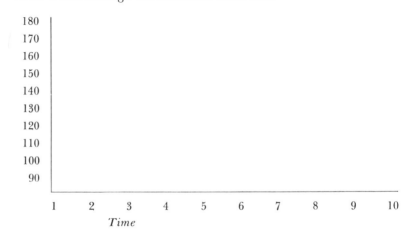

6. To illustrate the use of the preceding graph: A 16-year-old female field hockey player using the Morehouse formula from Statement 41 has a threshold heart rate of 147.0. If for the ten periods of interval training her HRs are: 114, 126. 138, 140, 144, 147, 162, 168, 156, and 162, how will she plot her heart rate response?

  This method would allow the participant to increase the work rate if the HR is too low or slow down if the HR is too high. Thus, it can be observed that our field hockey player is at or below her threshold rate for 6 of the 10 exercise bouts.

Teaching Methods

Performance Objectives

  The student should be able to monitor heart rate during a prescribed period of exercise and to plot this on a graph.

TABLE 8–3.   Conversion Table for 10-Second to One-Minute Heart Rate Test.

10-Sec *HR*	Min HR	10-Sec *HR*	Min HR
15	90	23	138
16	96	24	144
17	102	25	150
18	108	26	156
19	114	27	162
20	120	28	168
21	126	29	174
22	132	30	180

Teaching Hints
1. Statements 40 and 41 should be discussed prior to this statement.
2. Most of the hints are covered under procedures.

Discussion   1. Did you reach the appropriate level in all activities at all times? How did you adjust if the stress was too low or too high?
2. Does a sedentary middle aged adult need the same amount of physical stress as a well conditioned high school athlete?
3. If two people exercise together and one has a much higher average pulse rate (135 as compared to 110) than the other, what can you say about the physical fitness levels of the two people?

Materials   1. The two charts listed under Procedures.
2. A stopwatch or gym clock.

statement 43

> Cardiac output is directly proportional to the intensity of the exercise, is dependent upon the heart rate and stroke volume, and can be altered by cardiovascular training.

Introduction   It has been discussed previously that physically trained people are better able to deliver larger amounts of blood, oxygen, and fuel to the exercising muscles for the production of energy. One of the training adaptations in the cardiovascular system is an increased cardiac output. (The amount of blood pumped by the left ventricle of the heart per minute is termed cardiac output.) Cardiac output increases proportionately with the intensity of the work and is higher in trained persons for a given heart rate. For example, at rest the cardiac output of a human being is between 5 and 7 liters. This can increase up to 30 liters in a trained individual and 22 liters in an untrained person.

Stroke volume is the amount of blood pumped by the left ventricle of the heart per beat. This also is influenced by the state of training. A trained person will have an increased stroke volume both at rest and during maximal exercise.

This statement should allow the students to determine their own cardiac output and stroke volume while comparing these values to classmates at a variety of fitness levels.

Procedure   1. Cardiac output can be estimated easily by using the formula:

$$\text{Cardiac Output (Q)} = \frac{\text{VO}_2 \text{ in liters per minute}}{\text{A-V Difference (Table 8–4)}}$$

For example, a 20-year-old male predicts 2.5 L/min on the bicycle ergometer test (Statement 30). From Table 8–4 we estimate the arterial-venous (A-V) difference for 2.5 L to be 0.123; therefore we calculate the cardiac output (Q) to be 20 liters/min.

$$\text{Cardiac Output (Q)}$$

$$\frac{2.5\text{L}}{0.123} \qquad\qquad Q = 20 \text{ Liters/minute}$$

TABLE 8–4. Predicted Arterial Venous Difference.

VO₂ (ML/MIN)	ART-VEN. O₂ DIFF. (ML/ML)	VO₂ (ML/MIN)	ART-VEN. O₂ DIFF. (ML/ML)
250	0.045	2000	0.109
325	0.048	2200	0.115
400	0.050	2400	0.120
500	0.055	2600	0.125
600	0.060	2800	0.130
800	0.065	3000	0.135
1000	0.075	3200	0.139
1200	0.083	3400	0.143
1400	0.090	3600	0.146
1600	0.098	3800	0.150
1800	0.103		

From data of Rushmer as adapted by Benjamin Ricci in *Physiological Basis of Human Performance*. Philadelphia: Lea and Febiger, 1969, p. 267.

2. Stroke volume (SV) can be estimated by using the formula

$$SV = \frac{\text{Cardiac Output milliliters/min}}{\text{Heart Rate}} \qquad SV = \frac{Q}{HR}$$

For example, assume that the subject above had a cardiac output of 20 liters per minute during exercise. The formula calls for Q in ml/min or 20000. The heart rate is taken from the average of the fifth and sixth minute during the bicycle ergometer test (Statement 30).

$$\text{Stroke Volume (SV)} = \frac{20000}{142}$$

$$SV = 141 \text{ ml/stroke}$$

Teaching Methods

Performance Objective

The student should be able to calculate cardiac output and stroke volume based on the formulae given and information available.

Teaching Hints

1. The instructor must give the A-V difference information from the table provided.

2. Demonstrate a calculation of both Q and SV. It might save time if all the information, VO₂ (L/min), and heart rate are taken from Statement 30.

3. Qs and SVs might be listed on the board according to fitness categories with average scores for each determined. This would show the student how cardiac output is related to fitness levels.

Discussion   1. Do cardiac output and stroke volume partially account for improved fitness characteristics?

2. Is a high cardiac output correlated to high fitness levels?

3. Would a fit individual's heart react to exercise or an emergency more rapidly than that of an unfit person? Should firemen be in good categories of fitness?

statement 44

> Clothing has an effect upon body temperature and energy expenditure.

Introduction

Intense physical activity will increase the central or core temperature of the human body. Dissipation of this heat is important and is accomplished by the body in three ways: evaporation (sweating), convection (through the skin), and radiation (heat waves).

For each of these three methods to occur, internal heat must be transmitted from the central core of the body to the skin via the circulatory system. Consequently, a good barometer of the ability to transfer heat is the reaction of the cardiovascular system to alterations in the environment.

Exercise clothing must be carefully selected to aid in heat regulation. Some overzealous "exercise nuts" use rubber suits to sweat off extra pounds. Such stress, placed unnecessarily upon the cardiovascular system by improper clothing, may have a less than desirable effect.

Procedure

1. The subject should ride the bicycle ergometer for 5 minutes at 600 KPM.
2. A systolic blood pressure reading should be taken during the final minute of exercise. A skin thermometer should be strapped to the wrist to determine skin temperature.
3. After a short rest, the subject should dress in a rubber suit and take the test again.
4. Record the following data:

		Heart Rate					Pressure (Systolic)	Skin Temperature
	Rest	1	2	3	4	5		
Normal	___	__	__	__	__	__	_____	_____
Experimental	___	__	__	__	__	__	_____	_____

Teaching Methods

Performance Objective

The student should be able to record the skin temperature and cardiac response to exercise in two different conditions of dress.

Teaching Hints
1. This exercise should be conducted as a demonstration.
2. Select a student in good physical condition. The exercise bout with clothing will elevate the HR considerably.
3. A rubber suit is suggested for the experimental condition. Also, provide a hat and gloves.
4. Leave the blood pressure cuff on under the rubber suit. Remove the top of the suit quickly at the end of the exercise period and take the systolic blood pressure.
5. If a bicycle ergometer is unavailable, use a step test.

Discussion
1. What was the result of the experimental conditions?
2. What is the effect of improper clothing during exercise upon the cardiovascular system?
3. Why would this be undesirable for an overweight, out-of-shape middle-aged man or woman?
4. Should water be consumed during exercise?

Materials
1. Bicycle ergometer, heart rate conversion charts, stethoscope, blood pressure apparatus, a rubber suit, hat and gloves, and a skin thermometer.
2. A stethoscope, blood pressure apparatus, and skin thermometer can be purchased from the J. A. Preston Corp. 71 Fifth Ave., New York, N.Y. 10003.

statement 45

Impairment of insulin production can affect health.

Introduction A method to evaluate the normal metabolism of carbohydrate is to analyze the urine for carbohydrate content. In the nondiabetic population a large carbohydrate meal would signal the pancreas to release insulin to help in the carbohydrate metabolism. If insulin is unavailable, the blood sugar level will rapidly increase, resulting in an excess amount of glucose being filtered out into the urine. Consequently, a method to evaluate the individual's ability to metabolize glucose is to measure the level of sugar in the urine.

A glucose analysis of the urine is a standard procedure in most physical examinations. A positive test would indicate a possible alteration in insulin metabolism and could indicate a diabetic condition. It is estimated that 2.5 million known diabetics exist in the U.S. while another 2.5 million are undiagnosed. The sooner proper adjustments can be made in the diabetic, the less chance there will be of any serious long-range complications.

Procedure
1. Give each student a strip of glucose test tape.
2. Directions must be given to the students for the administration of the test. The directions will differ with the type of tape used.
3. Space should be provided on the lesson sheet to attach the test tape.

Teaching Methods

Performance Objective
The student should be able to assess whether or not sugar is present in the urine by use of the test tape provided.

Teaching Hints
1. A complete explanation must be given the student regarding the use of the tape. The students can use the tape at home, and then report the results to the class.
2. This statement can lead into a good discussion of diabetes and

weight control through diet and exercise. Overweight seems to be one predisposing factor to the onset of diabetes.

Discussion   1. Does the student show any trace of sugar in the urine? If so, how much?
2. Do you know any people with diabetes? Are they sick? Do they function normally? Can they exercise? Can they be treated with pills, diet, or injections? Can they get married and have children?
3. If you have diabetes in your family, what are your chances of developing this condition?

Materials   Test Tape. This can be purchased at any drug store. If the instructor conducts this statement at the appropriate time, some drug stores may provide tapes free during National Diabetes Week.

statement **46**

Relaxation techniques are easily learned and can be used to combat stress.

Introduction Our technological and highly structured society places great amounts of stress upon our various biological systems. Selye states that although we can adapt to minimal amounts of stress; over a long period of time continued stress can result in death.[1] Two possible methods for combating stress are presented through this statement: Jacobson's Relaxation Technique[2] and the practice of yoga.

Procedure 1. Have the students lie on mats. First, use Jacobson's Relaxation Technique (see Table 8–5). To assess the desired results, have the students take a pulse count immediately upon assuming the supine position. Again have a pulse count taken immediately upon the completion of the relaxation exercises. Record and average both heart rates.
2. Conduct some yoga exercises. Several good books are available on this topic.

Teaching Methods *Performance Objective*
    The student should be able to participate in two techniques that promote relaxation and help to relieve stress.

Teaching Hints
1. The students should be lying quietly on the mats during the Jacobson technique. The instructor will read the directions.
2. The yoga lesson is a bit more difficult unless the instructor has some previous experience.
3. Provide some appropriate yoga music. The music department in the school should be helpful. For the exercises, refer to any books on yoga which can be obtained at any library or bookstore.

---

[1] Hans Selye, *The Stress of Life* (New York: McGraw-Hill Book Co., 1956).

[2] E. Jacobson, *Progressive Relaxation* (Chicago: University of Chicago Press, 1956).

TABLE 8–5. Progressive Muscular Relaxation Technique.

1. Bend the right foot toward the face—let it go—bend it halfway—let it go—just barely bend it—let it go. Let the right foot go.

2. Bend the left foot toward the face—let it go—bend it halfway toward the face—let it go—just barely bend it—let it go. Let the left foot go. Let the right foot go.

3. Bend the right foot away from the face—let it go—just barely bend it—let it go. Let the right foot go.

4. Bend the left foot away from the face—let it go—just barely bend it—let it go. Let the left foot go. Let the right foot go.

5. Lift the right leg up—let it down—let it go. Lift the right leg up halfway—let it down—let it go. Lift the right leg up six inches—let it go—let the left foot go—let the right foot go.

6. Lift the left leg up—let it down—let it go—lift the left leg up halfway—let it down—let it go. Lift the left leg up six inches—let it down—let it go. Let the left leg go—let the right leg go—let the left foot go—let the right foot go.

7. Tighten up the gluteal muscles—let them go. Tighten them a little—let them go. Let the left leg go—let the right leg go.

8. Tighten the adominal muscles—let them go—tighten them just a little—let them go—let the right leg go—let the left leg go.

9. Arch the back—let it go—arch it just a little—let it go. Let the back muscles go—let the abdominal muscles go—let the right leg go—let the left leg go.

10. Tighten up the chest muscles—let them go—tighten them up just a little bit—let the chest muscles go—let the back muscles go—let the abdominal muscles go—let the right leg go—let the left leg go.

11. Tighten up the back muscles—let them go—tighten them up just a little bit—let them go—let the chest muscles go—let the abdominal muscles go—let the legs go.

12. Shrug the shoulders hard—let them go—shrug a little bit—let them go. Let the back go—let the chest go—let the abdomen go—let the legs go.

13. Tighten the right arm—let it go—tighten it a little—let it go. Let the shoulders go—let the back go—let the abdomen go—let the legs go.

14. Tighten the left arm—let it go—tighten it a little—let it go. Let the shoulders go—let the back go—let the abdomen go—let the legs go.

15. Take a deep breath—let it go—take a deep breath—let it go. Let the chest go, the back, the abdomen, the legs, the arms.

16. Raise the head—let it down—raise it a little—let it down—let the head go. Let the chest go, the back, the abdomen, the legs, the arms.

17. Close the jaws tightly—let them go—open the jaws wide—let them go—show the teeth—let it go—round the lips tightly—let them go—close the eyelids tightly—let them go. Let the whole body go.

By permission of E. Jacobson, *Progressive Relaxation*. Chicago: University of Chicago Press, 1956.

4. It would be more appropriate to have a certified instructor in the Jacobson Method and one in Yoga to teach this statement if they are available.

Discussion

1. How did you feel after using Jacobson's technique?
2. What was your heart rate prior to the technique? After the program? What was the group average before and after?
3. How did you feel after the yoga exercises?
4. What are the differences between American exercise techniques and games and yoga?
5. What component of fitness may be developed by yoga?
6. What biological system can be influenced by yoga?

Materials

1. Jacobson's Relaxation Technique.
2. Phonograph and appropriate yoga music.
3. Books on yoga exercises.

statement 47

> The physical and emotional response to stress is due to hormonal secretion and is largely under neural control.

Introduction The "flight or fight" response to stress is a universal experience. An immediate indicator of the reaction to stress is the heart rate. Several hormones, primarily the catecholamines (epinephrine and norepinephrine), cortisol, growth hormone, antidiuretic hormone, and glucogen are secreted to mobilize the energy and energy support systems for both physical and emotional stress.

The endocrinological syndrome of physical activity involves five time partitions: anticipation of the forthcoming experience, initial stage of exercise, adaptation to the exercise, exhaustion (optional: depends upon the nature of the stress), and recovery from the exercise. The student should think in terms of these stages while completing several of the exercise statements.

Procedure
1. Establish a resting heart rate for each student as each lies on a mat.
2. Present a variety of emotional and physical stress conditions to the student. Between each stress application the student should lie on a mat to reduce the heart rate to resting levels (immediately following the stress and for two minutes thereafter).
3. Some suggested emotional stress conditions (remember that a resting HR must be taken prior to each stress application):
   a. A loud scream or horn blast while the student is resting on a mat with the eyes closed.
   b. Without the use of pencil and paper, have student very rapidly add a column of figures verbally presented.
   c. Present a gruesome picture of an automobile accident, war scene, starving children, etc.
   d. Present tactile stimuli such as raw eggs, noodles, cold cream, etc., to blindfolded student.
   e. Present such unpleasant pungent odors as ammonia, spoiled food, etc.
4. Some suggested physical stress conditions:
   a. There is a variety of physical tests that can be administered (such as the Astrand Bike Test, PWC-170, the Harvard Step Test, etc.).

217

b. Measure the effect of various postures—such as lying, sitting, standing—on HR.

Teaching Methods

Performance Objective

Student should be able to perceive increased heart rate as an indicator of stress.

Teaching Hints

1. Sitting or lying on a mat will make the emotional stress conditions effective. In both emotional and physical stress conditions, timing is important. Allow enough time between the presentation of the various stimuli.
2. Have students work in groups of two. Blindfolds can be provided.
3. Response charts and graphs should be developed, such as the following.

STRESS CHART

		Stress Heart Rate		
Resting Heart Rate	*Stress Condition*	*1st Min.*	*2nd Min.*	*3rd Min.*
1.				
2.				
3.				
4.				

Discussion

1. Which type of stress condition produced the greatest heart rate: physical or emotional?
2. Do all people react the same way to stress?
3. Can heart rate be reduced consciously? Can increased heart rate be prevented in response to stress stimuli?
4. How did you respond during the five stages of the exercise syndrome as described?

Materials

Dependent upon the instructor. Suggestions are made under Procedures and Teaching Methods.

statement 48

Cardiac metabolism is oxygen-dependent and can be an indicator of heart disease.

Introduction

Use of oxygen by the heart is called myocardial oxygen consumption (MVO_2). This can be estimated by the formula given below. It has been discovered that people with heart trouble consume more oxygen during exercise owing to a decreased efficiency of the myocardium. The so-called "double product" of systolic blood pressure and heart rate has been used to estimate MVO_2.[1] Studies indicate improvement in this condition with training in heart patients.

The students should be able to determine myocardial oxygen uptake using the formula and previously gathered information.

Procedure

1. The formula for determining Myocardial Oxygen Consumption (MVO_2):

$$MVO_2 = \text{Systolic Blood Pressure} \times \text{Heart Rate}$$

The systolic blood pressure and heart rate information will be used from Statement 49. If the subject mentioned in Statement 43 has a systolic blood pressure of 180 mmHg and a heart rate of 142 during the final minute of the bicycle ergometer test, then the MVO_2 can be calculated as follows:

$$MVO_2 = 180 \text{ mmHg} \times 142$$

$$MVO_2 = 255.6 \text{ ml } O_2/\text{min}$$

Teaching Methods

Performance Objective

The student should be able to determine the myocardial oxygen consumption using the formula and previously gathered information.

[1] D. T. Redwood, D. R. Rosing, and S. E. Epstein, "Circulatory and Symptomatic Effects of Physical Training in Patients with Coronary-Artery Disease and Angina Pectoris," *New England Journal of Medicine*, 286 (1972), 959–65. See also K. Kitamura, C. R. Jorgensen, F. L. Gobel, H. L. Taylor, and Y. Wang, "Hemodynamic Correlates of Myocardial Oxygen Consumption during Upright Exercise," *Journal of Applied Physiology*, 32 (1972), 516–22.

Teaching Hint

The formula is straightforward. Unfortunately, standards have not been established yet relating workload, HR, blood pressure, and possible coronary heart disease.

Discussion

1. What factors might account for lessening MVO_2 during exercise?
2. Would training influence any of these factors?
3. Which man would be most likely to have a problem?

Subject	Blood Pressure	Heart Rate	MVO_2
A	180	135	—
B	225	129	—
C	170	150	—
D	200	165	—

Materials   The given formula and the data are from the bicycle ergometer test.

statement 49

> Hypertension is one of the possible causative factors in cardiovascular disease.

Introduction   John Merrill, M.D., describes blood pressure as follows:

> Blood flow through the normal vascular bed may be thought of as a system in which pulsatile flow occurs in a series of elastic tubes. The larger tubes, represented by the arteries, gradually decrease in caliber through the arterioles to the capillaries and similarly decrease the magnitude of each pulsation until within the capillaries the flow becomes steady. In this system the pulsating force is provided by the contraction of the left ventricle, the elasticity by the walls of the arteries, and the major portion of the resistance of flow by the arterial bed. The pressure produced at the peak of ventricular contraction in the elastic system is represented by the systolic blood pressure, and the total resting resistance of the system in ventricular diastole by the diastolic pressure.[1]

High blood pressure, or hypertension, is one of the possible causative factors in cardiovascular disease. Proper screening is necessary to identify potential problems in the cardiovascular system. Treatment of high blood pressure generally involves drug and/or diet therapy.

The AMA has recently established standards for hypertension and is suggesting a nationwide screening program.[2]

$$\frac{140 \text{ mmHg}}{90 \text{ mmHg}} \qquad \text{No further attention necessary}$$

$$\frac{160 \text{ mmHg}}{95 \text{ mmHg}} \qquad \text{Needs immediate referral}$$

If diastolic blood pressure exceeds 105 mmHg, immediate referral is indicated.

[1] John P. Merrill "Hypertension Vascular Disease," in *Principles of Internal Medicine*, 5th ed. (New York: McGraw-Hill Book Co., 1966), p. 703.

[2] "Hypertension Screening: Defining the Problem, Setting Priorities," *JAMA*, 233 (1973), 901–902.

Procedure   Have the blood pressure taken. If considered abnormal according to the above standards, wait 30 seconds and repeat.

Teaching Methods

Performance Objective
    The student should be able to take blood pressure readings.

Teaching Hint
    The instructor should train one or two class member to administer the blood pressure test. If time and equipment permits, the entire class can be taught this technique for a much better understanding of this very important examination method.

Discussion
1. What are some of the factors leading to high blood pressure?
2. What are the effects of training in the normalization of blood pressure?
3. Should a person with serious hypertension begin an exercise program? What happens to blood pressure with exercise?

Materials   Blood pressure apparatus and stethoscope.

statement 50

Some of the factors leading to arteriosclerotic heart disease may be controlled by the individual.

Introduction Arteriosclerotic heart disease (AHD) is a condition involving many factors. Paffenbarger states:

> Only by expanding our efforts in the direction of primary prevention are we likely to make major progress toward control of heart disease. The secondary approach of waiting to intervene until disease is overt is much less promising. Programs should aim for control of high-risk factors early in life. The disease that underlies the coronary attack of middle age begins in childhood.[1]

John Boyer has developed a Cardiac Risk Index (see Table 8–6) based on eight factors.[2] The student should take the test and discuss the questions in the Discussion section.

Procedure 1. The student should complete the Cardiac Risk Index in Table 8–6.

Teaching Methods

Performance Objective

The student should be able to determine cardiac risk by comparong scores to those values in Table 8–7.

Teaching Hints

1. Statements 6, 30, 33, 48, and 49 should be completed prior to using the Cardiac Risk Index.
2. This statement is best completed in class under the instructor's supervision. Factor 6 in the Cardiac Risk Index—cholesterol or percentage of fat in the diet—is difficult to determine accurately; only an estimation can be made for the purpose of completing this Statement. The usual American diet contains about 30 percent animal fat, and high school and college students of normal weight and

---

[1]Ralph S. Paffenbarger, Jr., "Prevention of Heart Disease," *Postgraduate Medicine*, 51 (January 1972), pp. 74.

[2]John L. Boyer, M.D., Director of San Diego State University Exercise Physiology Laboratory, San Diego, California.

TABLE 8-6. Cardiac Risk Index.

	10 to 20	21 to 30	31 to 40	41 to 50	51 to 60	61 to 70 and over
1. Age	No. 1	2	3	4	6	8
2. *Heredity*	No known history of heart disease 1	1 relative with cardiovascular disease over 60 2	2 relatives with cardiovascular disease over 60 3	1 relative with cardiovascular disease under 60 4	2 relatives with cardiovascular disease under 60 6	3 relatives with cardiovascular disease under 60. 8
3. *Weight*	More than 5 lbs. below standard weight 0	Standard weight 1	5–20 lbs. overweight 2	21–35 lbs. overweight 3	36–50 lbs. overweight 5	51–65 lbs. overweight 7
4. *Tobacco Smoking*	Nonuser 0	Cigar and/or pipe 1	10 cigarettes or less a day 2	20 cigarettes a day 3	30 cigarettes a day 5	40 cigarettes a day or more 8
5. *Exercise*	Intensive occupational and recreational exertion 1	Moderate occupational and recreational exertion 2	Sedentary work and intense recreational exertion 3	Sedentary occupational and moderate recreational exertion 5	Sedentary work and light recreational exertion 6	Complete lack of all exercise 8

By permission of John L. Boyer, Director of San Diego University Exercise Physiology Laboratory, San Diego, California.

TABLE 8-6. Continued

6. *Cholesterol or % fat in diet*	Cholesteral below 180 mg. Diet contains no animal or solid fats [1]	Cholesterol 181–205 mg. Diet contains 10% animal or solid fats [2]	Cholesterol 206–230 mg. Diet contains 20% animal or solid fats [3]	Cholesterol 231–255 mg. Diet contains 30% animal or solid fats [4]	Cholesterol 256–280 mg. Diet contains 40% animal or solid fats [5]	Cholesterol 281–330 mg. Diet contains 50% animal or solid fats [7]
7. *Blood Pressure*	100 upper reading [1]	120 upper reading [2]	140 upper reading [3]	160 upper reading [4]	180 upper reading [6]	200 or over upper reading [8]
8. *Sex*	Female [1]	Female over 45 [2]	Male [3]	Bald Male [4]	Bald short male [6]	Bald short stocky male [7]

Total Score: _____

225

TABLE 8–7. Cardiovascular Disease Risk Index Scoring Table.

Group I	6 to 11	= very low risk
Group II	12 to 17	= low risk
Group III	18 to 25	= average risk
Group IV	26 to 32	= high risk
Group V	33 to 42	= dangerous risk
Group VI	42 to 60	= extremely dangerous risk

average somatotype have cholesterol levels of less than 200 mg percent. However, an overweight student or a mature mesomorph could be as high as 250 mg percent.

3. Complete the questions under discussion.

Discussion

1. List your risk category.
2. Which factor was the highest?
3. What can be done about your two highest risk factors?
4. List someone you know who has recently had a heart attack. What risk factors does he or she seem to have?

Materials   The Cardiac Risk Index and Scoring Table.

statement 51

> Certain patterns of behavior may increase the possibilities of heart disease.

Introduction   Friedman and Rosenman reported that "intensely ambitious men who drive themselves in work or play and race to meet deadlines are particularly susceptible to angina and coronary occlusions."[1] Their study involved two selected groups of subjects with opposite emotional attitudes. Group A was made up of men characterized by relatively intense drive, aggressiveness, ambitiousness, competitiveness, a pressure to pit themselves against the clock, and a pressure for getting things done. Group B was composed of men who, though equally serious, were more easy-going in manner, seldom became impatient, and were apt to take more time to enjoy leisure; they were not driven by the clock, not preoccupied with social achievements, were less competitive, even speaking in a more modulated style. Surprisingly, Type As were found to go to bed earlier than Type Bs, who tended to be interested in things irrelevant to their careers and sit up late, or simply socialize. Most people are mixtures of Type A and Type B. The findings indicated that coronary heart disease occurred much more frequently in Type A than in Type B people. In fact, in the population studied, 29 sudden cardiac deaths were of the Type A variety, while there were only 2 of Type B; 6 deaths were undetermined.

Procedure   The student should answer the questions in Table 8–8.

Teaching Methods

Performance Objective

   The student should be able to determine a Type A or Type B behavior pattern by completing Table 8–8.

---

[1]M. Friedman and R. H. Rosenman, "Association of Specific Overt Behavior Pattern with Blood and Cardiovascular Findings," *Journal of American Medical Association*, 169 (1959), 1286–96. See also M. Friedman, J. H. Manwaring, R. H. Sesenman, G. Donlon, P. Ortega, and S. M. Grube, "Instantaneous and Sudden Deaths, *Journal of the American Medical Association*, 225 (1973), 1319–28.

TABLE 8–8. Cardiac Risk Behavioral Pattern Questionnaire.

Respond to the following questions with YES *or* NO *answers.*

1. I have an intense sustained drive to get ahead.	*Yes*___ *No*___
2. I'm anxious to reach my goals, but I'm uncertain what those goals are.	*Yes*___ *No*___
3. I feel a need to compete and win.	*Yes*___ *No*___
4. I have a persistent desire for recognition.	*Yes*___ *No*___
5. I always seem to be involved in too many things at once.	*Yes*___ *No*___
6. I'm always racing the clock, constantly on edge, have deadlines.	*Yes*___ *No*___
7. I have a need to speed things up, get things done faster.	*Yes*___ *No*___
8. I'm extraordinarily alert mentally and physically.	*Yes*___ *No*___
Total	___ ___

By permission of M. Friedman and R.H. Rosenman from "Association of Specific Overt Behavior Patterns with Blood and Cardiovascular Findings," *Journal of the American Medical Association*, 169 (1959), 1286–96.

Teaching Hint

The students should complete Table 8–8 prior to reading the introductory section for this statement.

Discussion   1. What is your predominate behavior pattern?

2. List two of the YES responses, and state how you can alter these.

Glossary

A   *Adaptation*   The process of adjusting to stress

    ATP (Adenosine Tri Phosphate)   A molecule that provides the immediate energy for muscular contraction

    Aerobic   The generation of energy coupled to the utilization of oxygen

    Agility   The ability to change directions quickly

    Aging   The gradual loss of the ability to respond to the environment, the loss accompanied by an increase in an incidence of disease and probability of death

    Anaerobic   The generation of energy without coupling to the utilization of oxygen

    Arteriosclerosis   Loss of elasticity or hardening of the artery

B   *Balance*   The process of maintaining postural equilibrium

    Basal Metabolic Rate (BMR)   The amount of oxygen needed to sustain the least amount of bodily function

    Biological Awareness   An understanding of the body and how the body responds to the demands of the environment

    Body Composition   The components of the body divided into lean body mass, fat, and total body water

    Body Fat   The portion of the body that is composed of fatty tissue; usually expressed as a percentage of body weight

Body Image   The manner in which a person envisions his or her body

C   *Calorie*   A unit of energy usually referred to in nutritional studies

Carbohydrate   A classification of food that includes sugars and starches

Cardiac Output   The volume of blood pumped by the heart in one minute

Cardiorespiratory   Usually referred to as the integrated function of the lungs and heart

Cholesterol   A fat-like substance found in all animal tissues and fluids

Circuit Training   A series of exercises where the participant performs prescribed activities based on any combination of time, sets, and repetitions

Central Nervous System (CNS)   The neural system composed of the brain and the spinal cord

Concentric Contraction   The shortening of a muscle

Coordination   The act of the body working in harmony in a smooth way

Coronary Thrombosis   A blood clot in the coronary artery usually resulting in death of cardiac tissue

Creatine Phosphate   A molecule used by the body to regenerate ATP

D   *Diastolic Blood Pressure*   The blood pressure during the relaxation of the heart

Dynamic Contraction   Muscle contraction resulting in movement

E   *Eccentric Contraction*   The lengthening of a muscle against a resistance

Ectomorph   The component of the body characterized by linearity and skinnyness

Electrocardiograph   The recording of the electrical activity of the heart

Endomorph   The component of the body characterized by a large amount of body fat, roundness, and softness

Endurance   The ability to exercise for long periods of time

Energy Balance   An equilibrium between food intake and energy expenditure

Energy expenditure   Energy utilization measured in calories

Exercise   A nonresting state of the body; it can be classified according to speed of movement, resistance to movement, and duration of activity

Exercise Intensity Threshold (EIT)   The levels of exercise above which there will be an improvement in edurance fitness

F   *Fatigue*   The inability to continue an exercise

Flexibility   The full range of motion at a joint or series of joints

G *Glucose* The common form of carbohydrate usually referred to as sugar

Glycogen A storage form of carbohydrate found in body tissues

Graded Exercise Test (GET) A progressive exercise test to assess the functional capacity of the body

H *Hormone* A chemical substance transported via the blood to a target organ resulting in a specific reaction

Hypertension A pathologically elevated resting systolic blood pressure above 160

Hypertrophy Enlargement of a tissue

I *Ideal Body Weight* The desired body weight for a given body structure

Immediate Energy Sources The chemicals in the muscle available for immediate energy release

Isometric Contraction Contraction of a muscle against a resistance without resulting movement

K *KiloGram Meter (KGM)* A unit of work; the movement of a kilogram over a distance of one meter

KiloPond Meter (KPM) A unit of measure on the bicycle ergometer; the amount of force required to accelerate a mass of 1 kilogram 1 meter per sec. per sec.

L *Lactate* The end product of the nonoxidative utilization of carbohydrate

Lean Body Weight A component of body composition that excludes body fat

M *Maximal Heart Rate* The highest obtainable heart rate; usually age dependent

Maximal Oxygen Consumption The maximal amount of oxygen utilized per unit of time, usually considered to be the best indicator of endurance fitness (ml/kg/min)

Mesomorph The component of the body characterized by large amounts of muscle

Mitochondria The structure in the body responsible for oxygen utilization and aerobic energy production

Motor Unit A motor nerve and those muscle fibers innervated by that nerve

Myocardial Infarction The death of cardiac tissue resulting from coronary insufficiency

Myocardial Oxygen Consumption The use of oxygen by the heart, may be estimated by multiplying the heart rate by the systolic blood pressure

N   *Negative Energy Balance*   An energy expenditure level that is less than the level of food intake

Neuromuscular   The integrated function of the nerve and muscle

Nonoxidative Energy Sources   Those chemicals capable of supplying energy without the utilization of oxygen

O   *Obese*   A percentage of body fat above 39 percent

Overload Principle   The application of a suitable stress to a system, the stress being beyond that normally encountered

Overweight   A body weight above the height-weight standards based on body frame

Oxidative Energy Sources   Those chemicals capable of supplying energy coupled to the utilization ot oxygen

Oxygen Consumption   The amount of oxygen being used by the body

P   *Physical Fitness*   The functional capacity of how the body responds to the demands of the environment

Positive Energy Balance   An energy expenditure level that is greater than the level of food intake

Power   The application of a force per unit of time

Protein   A classification of chemicals made up of amino acids, most commonly found as enzymes, contractile and structural elements of tissues

R   *Reaction Time*   The time necessary to react to a stimulus

Recommended Daily Allowance (RDA)   The required daily intake of foodstuffs, vitamins and minerals for adequate nutrition

RM   The maximum number of repetitions that can be performed in a specific person at a specific point in time

S   *Somatotype*   A system of characterizing the components of body physique

Specificity of Exercise   A specific exercise results in a specific response in a specific person

Specificity of Training   A specific exercise regimen will result in a specific adaptation within the body

Speed of Movement   The quickness of movement of the body or of specific body parts

Spirokinesis   The fundamental veering tendency in man

Static Contraction   Contraction of a muscle against a resistance without resulting in movement

Strength   The maximum application of force for a specified activity

Stress   Those outside forces acting on the body that, if continued, will result in adaptations

Stroke Volume   The volume of blood pumped by the heart per stroke

Systolic Blood Pressure   The blood pressure during the contraction phase of the heart beat

T   *Training*   The process of adapting to daily exercise sessions

Triglycerides   The form of storage and blood transport of fat

U   *Ultrastructure*   The structure of a tissue observed through a micro-scope

V   *Vascularization*   The blood supply to a tissue

Vital Capacity   The volume of gas which can be exhaled by a maximal voluntary effort following a full inspiration

Vitamin   A classification of chemicals that are necessary for normal metabolism

General Bibliography

ASTRAND, P. O. and K. RODAHL, *Textbook of Work Physiology*. New York: McGraw-Hill, Inc., 1970.

BARNEY, V. S., C. C. HIRST, and C. R. JENSON, *Conditioning Exercises*. St. Louis, Missouri: The C. V. Mosby Co., 1969.

BEHNKE, A. R. and J. H. WILMORE, *Evaluation and Regulation of Body Build and Composition*. Englewood Cliffs, New Jersey: Prentice-Hall, Inc., 1974.

BERGER, R. A., *Conditioning for Man*. Boston: Allyn and Bacon, Inc., 1973.

CORBIN, C. B., L. J. DOWELL, R. LINDSEY, and H. TOLSON, *Concepts in Physical Education*. Dubuque, Iowa: William C. Brown, 1970.

DE VRIES, H. A., *Physiology of Exercise for P. E. and Athletics*, 2nd edition. Dubuque, Iowa: William C. Brown Co., 1973.

EDINGTON, D. W. and V. R. EDGERTON, *Biology of Activity*. Boston: Houghton-Mifflin Co., 1976.

FALLS, H. B., ed. *Exercise Physiology*. New York: Academic Press, 1968.

FALLS, H. B., E. L. WALLIS, and G. A. LOGAN, *Foundations of Conditioning*. New York: Academic Press, 1970.

FLEISHMAN, E. A. *The Structure and Measurement of Physical Fitness*. Englewood Cliffs, New Jersey: Prentice-Hall, Inc., 1963.

FOX, E. L. and D. K. MATTHEWS, *Interval Training*. Philadelphia: W. B. Saunders, Co., 1974.

FRANKS, D. B. and H. DEUTSCH, *Evaluation Performance in P. E.* New York: Academic Press, Inc., 1973.

GOLDING, L. A. and R. R. BOS, *Scientific Foundations of P. E. and Fitness Programs*, 2nd ed. Minneapolis, Minnesota: Burgess Publishing Co., 1970.

HOCKEY, P. V., *Physical Fitness*. St. Louis, Missouri: The C. V. Mosby Co., 1973.

JENSEN, C. R. and A. G. FISHER, *Scientific Basis of Athletic Conditioning*. Philadelphia: Lea and Febiger, Inc., 1972.

JOKL, E. and P. JOKL, *The Physiological Basis of Athletic* Records. Springfield, Illinois: Charles C. Thomas Publishers, 1968.

JOHNSON, B. L. and J. K. NELSON, *Practical Measurement for Evaluation in P. E.* Minneapolis, Minn.: Burgess Publishing Co., 1969.

JOHNSON, P. and D. STOLBURG, *Conditioning*. Englewood Cliffs, N.J.: Prentice-Hall, Inc., 1971.

KARPOVICH, P. V. and W. E. SINNING, *Physiology of Muscular Activity*, 7th edition. Philadelphia, Pa.: W. B. Saunders Co., 1971.

KASCH, F. W. and J. L. BOYER, *Adult Fitness: Principles and Practices*. Palo Alto, Calif.: National Press Books, 1968.

KIPHUTH, R. *How To Be Fit*. New Haven, Conn.: Yale University Press, 1963.

KLAFS, C. E. and M. J. LYON, *The Female Athlete*. St. Louis, Missouri: The C. V. Mosby Co., 1973.

LARSON, L. A. and H. MICHELMAN, *International Guide to Fitness and Health*. New York: Crown Publishers, Inc., 1973.

MATTHEWS, D. K. *Measurement in P. E.* Philadelphia, Pa.: W. B. Saunders Co., 1973.

MAYER, J. *Overweight*. Englewood Cliffs, New Jersey: Prentice-Hall, Inc., 1967.

MOREHOUSE, L. E. and A. T. MILLER, *Exercise Physiology*, 5th edition. St. Louis, Missouri: The C. V. Mosby Co., 1967.

MORGAN, W. P. *Ergogenic Aids and Muscular Performance*. New York: Academic Press, Inc., 1972.

PARNELL, WILLIAM, *Behavior and Physiques: An Introduction to Practical Applied Somatology*. London: Arnold Pub., Ltd., 1958.

PEEBLER, J. R. and D. W. E. BAIRD, *Controlled Exercise for Physical Fitness*. Springfield, Ill.: Charles C. Thomas Publishers, 1962.

RARICK, G. L., Editor, *Physical Activity, Human Growth and Development*. New York: Academic Press, Inc., 1973.

RICCI, B. *Physiological Basis of Human Performance*. Philadelphia, Pa.: Lea and Febiger, Co., 1967.

ROBB, D. *The Dynamics of Motor Skill Acquisition*. Englewood Cliffs, New Jersey: Prentice-Hall, Inc., 1972.

SAFRIT, M. J. *Evaluation in Physical Education*. Englewood Cliffs, New Jersey: Prentice-Hall, Inc., 1973.

SCOTT, G. M. and E. FRENCH, *Measurement and Evaluation in Physical Education*. Dubuque, Iowa: William C. Brown Publishers, 1959.

SHEEHAN, T. J., *An Introduction to the Evaluation of Measurement Data in P. E.* Reading, Massachusetts: Addison-Wesley Publishing Co., 1971.

SHEPARD, R. J., *Endurance Fitness*. Toronto: University of Toronto Press, 1969.

SHEPARD, R. J., ed., *Frontiers of Fitness*. Springfield, Illinois: Charles C. Thomas Publishers, 1971.

STEINHAUS, A. H., *Toward an Understanding of Health and Physical Education*, Dubuque, Iowa: William C. Brown Co., 1963.

SWENGROS, G. with J. MONTELEONE, *Fitness with Glen Swengros*. New York: Hawthorn Books, Inc., 1971.

VAN HUSS, W. D., R. R. NIEMEYRR, H. W. OLSON, and J. A. FRIEDRICH, *Physical Activity in Modern Living*, 2nd ed., Englewood Cliffs, New Jersey: Prentice-Hall, Inc., 1969.

VITALE, F., *Individualized Fitness Programs*. Englewood Cliffs, New Jersey: Prentice-Hall, Inc., 1973.

WILLGOOSE, C. E., *Evaluation in Health Education and Physical Education*. New York: McGraw-Hill, Inc., 1961.

Index